Continence care pathways

Continence care pathways

Valerie Bayliss

RN, MSc

Rachel Locke

BA(hons), MA, PhD

Elizabeth Salter

RN, RM

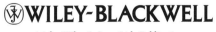

WILEY-BLACKWELL

A John Wiley & Sons, Ltd., Publication

This edition first published 2009
© 2009 John Wiley & Sons

Wiley-Blackwell is an imprint of John Wiley and Sons, formed by the merger of
Wiley's global Scientific, Technical and Medical business with Blackwell Publishing.

Registered office
John Wiley & Sons Ltd, The Atrium, Southern Gate, Chichester, West Sussex,
PO19 8SQ, United Kingdom

Editorial office
John Wiley & Sons Ltd, The Atrium, Southern Gate, Chichester, West Sussex,
PO19 8SQ, United Kingdom

For details of our global editorial offices, for customer services and for information
about how to apply for permission to reuse the copyright material in this book please
see our website at www.wiley.com/wiley-blackwell.

The right of the author to be identified as the author of this work has been asserted in
accordance with the Copyright, Designs and Patents Act 1988.

Library of Congress Cataloging-in-Publication Data

Bayliss, Valerie, 1954–
    Continence care pathways / Valerie Bayliss, Rachel Locke, Elizabeth Salter.
      p. ; cm.
    Includes bibliographical references and index.
    ISBN 978-0-470-06143-5 (pbk. : alk. paper)   1. Urinary incontinence–Nursing.
2. Faecal incontinence–Nursing.   3. Evidence-based nursing.   4. Critical path
analysis.   I. Locke, Rachel, 1967–   II. Salter, Elizabeth, 1947–   III. Title.
    [DNLM: 1. Urinary Incontinence–nursing. 2. Critical Pathways. 3. Faecal
Incontinence–nursing. WJ 146 B358c 2009]
    RC921.I5.B39 2009
    616.6'2–dc22

                                                                        2008049832

A catalogue record for this book is available from the British Library.

Set in 11/13 pt Minion by Aptara® Inc., New Delhi, India
Printed and bound in Singapore by Fabulous Printers Pte Ltd

1   2009

Contents

Dedication

We dedicate this book to Kevin, Paul, Sean, Anna, James and William and thank them for their patience and support during its formation.

About the authors

Valerie Bayliss RN, MSc
Clinical Nurse Specialist, Hampshire Primary Care Trust
Basingstoke, Hampshire

Rachel Locke BA(hons), MA, PhD
Research Officer, University of Winchester
Winchester, Hampshire

Elizabeth Salter RN, RM
Clinical Nurse Specialist, Swindon PCT (retired)
Bradenstoke, Wiltshire

Biographical information

All three authors contributed to the development of *Continence Care Pathways* and the dissemination of the findings through, amongst other things, a series of articles for the *British Journal of Nursing*. Valerie Bayliss and Liz Salter have worked as clinical nurse specialists in the area of continence care for the last 30 years. Dr Rachel Locke works as an academic researcher and carries out university-based and independent research.

Foreword

Written by the team that developed the original concept of bladder and bowel care pathways in the United Kingdom, this book provides a wealth of detail on how to assess, treat and manage a person with either or both of these conditions. Bladder and Bowel Dysfunction is notoriously the poor relation in all care delivery with audit undertaken by the Royal College of Physicians (Wagg *et al.*, 2005) demonstrating that incontinence inevitably results in the provision of a pad or catheter being the first line rather than end of line care. These pathways, which have been adopted throughout the United Kingdom by numerous bladder and bowel care specialist services, illustrate a proactive and interesting way of assessing patients in order to ensure that the patient actually gets the care they deserve, that is care where a pad or catheter is not the first option. The authors should be congratulated for writing this book. They have already illustrated by their development of the pathways that they have a real feel for bladder and bowel care. This book will ensure that their dream and enthusiasm is shared and, hopefully, copied. I have been nagging the authors to write up their work for a number of years and to see it come to fruition is brilliant. I hope that you enjoy reading the book as much as I have. I also hope that you take away something new from it in order to continue to develop your own practice and to make you think of how you can move the world of continence care on as much as the authors have in order to change the way our speciality is perceived.

Amanda Wells
Professional Executive Committee member, Clinical Lead for Cancer (Devon Primary Care Trust) and Consultant Nurse/Head of Department, Integrated Bladder and Bowel Care, Devon Primary Care Trust.

Preface

This book has been written for qualified nurses who have attained level three (degree) in the Research and Evidence-based Practice module. This could include district nurses, health visitors, midwives, psychiatric nurses, learning disability nurses, practice nurses and nurses caring for older people. Its aim is to improve care for patients with continence problems.

Incontinence has an enormous impact on the quality of a patient's life. It is a distressing condition for both the patients and their families, and one that can be cured or improved. Proper assessment and management of the problem is highlighted in a succession of policy documents, starting with *Good Practice in Continence Services* (Department of Health, 2000) and that appearing in the *NHS Next Stage Review: Our Vision for Primary and Community Care*, which requires that the evidence base for continence care pathways is reviewed to help to 'free up more time for direct patient care, and improve quality and patient outcomes' (Department of Health, 2008).

Care pathways are an evidence-based method of assessing and delivering care that put the patient at the centre. They can be used to provide high-quality care that is robust. They are dynamic, flexible tools that promote continence and provide information for health care professionals, patients and carers.

This book explains why the authors embarked upon the process of changing the way patients are assessed. It goes on to describe a set of suggested statements that could be utilised by users to design their own pathways for specific client groups. By involving the patient in the development of the pathways, communication is enhanced. How this is done is also discussed and illustrated in this book.

The authors intend that, by using this handbook, the reader will be empowered to develop and apply continence care pathways themselves.

We would like to thank some professional colleagues for their help and encouragement in writing the book. Specifically, thanks go to Rosie Richardson (RN, HV Cert.) for her contribution on communicating with patients in Chapter 2 and Mandy Wells for writing the foreword, her comments on a draft manuscript and for allowing us to use the Algorithm for Faecal Incontinence in Chapter 6. Grateful thanks also go to Sue Hallett for her helpful comments.

Chapter 1

An overview of continence care and the case for care pathways

Good-quality continence care can enhance the lives of people who suffer from this symptom. There has been a revolution in continence care starting towards the end of the last century and continuing into this one that recognises that continence problems are symptoms of an underlying disorder which may be primarily due to bladder or bowel dysfunction or, secondarily, to systemic disease processes. Prior to this, incontinence was simply managed with patient, bed or chair protection and patients were often deemed lazy or difficult. New research into diagnostics, treatments, therapies and lifestyles is regularly published and patients benefit from access to specialist advice and clinics. Many people are now able to maintain a high quality of life and there are even research-based, quality-of-life questionnaires that can validate this.

However, despite guidance there is little mandatory provision, which has led to inequitable service provision. The overall cost of continence care and management is set to rise substantially, as demographic changes affect service provision. In 2008 incontinence cost European health care systems and society £13 billion annually. This figure comes from a worldwide review of health economics literature relating to incontinence by Professor Rosanna Tarricone, health economist at the Centre for Research on Health Care Management at Bocconi University in Italy (Pountney, 2008).

The total expenditure for the United Kingdom is approximately 120th of the cost of the NHS (as at the year 2000) (Getliffe and

Dolman, 2003). This does not take into account the hidden cost associated with the psychological consequences of the condition, the costs of informal care, the ineffectiveness and inefficiency of some delivery systems and the inappropriateness of using inpatient care for individuals with incontinence.

This chapter seeks to look at the influences which have provoked such changes and details the changes to the traditional role of the nurse. The implications for nurses in continence care and the fact that their extended role has meant increased pressure on time and resources will also be explored. The chapter then goes on to discuss whether quality continence care may be less of a health care priority in the NHS, and considers some of the issues that this raises. The last section in this chapter describes care pathways and the benefits of their use.

Main policy documents

The first major document to bring continence care to the forefront was *Good Practice in Continence Services* (Department of Health, 2000). This document states that prompt, high-quality and comprehensive continence services are an integral part of the NHS. A review was set up in 1998, but it was an Audit Commission report (1999) – which said that district nurses were focusing on managing the problem of incontinence rather than treating it, despite it being a highly treatable condition – that did much to prompt the drawing-up of guidelines. These guidelines were later enshrined by the Department of Health (2000). However, there seemed at that time to be no political will to endorse the report's contents. A Royal College of Nursing survey showed that only 8% of Trusts were implementing one of the main recommendations, that of establishing a director of continence services in each Primary Care Trust (PCT), some years after the guidelines were published (Thomas, 2007). In 2001 the *National Service Framework for Older People* (Department of Health, 2001a) gave teeth to the guidelines by setting targets for having an integrated continence service in place by April 2004. However, subsequent audit showed that, in the majority of cases, this deadline had not been met (Wagg, 2004).

Nevertheless, the guidelines were successful in moving continence up the agenda both locally and nationally, and further papers were published shortly afterwards. Arguably, one of the most used was *Essence of Care* (Department of Health, 2001). The aim of this document was to improve the quality of the fundamental and essential aspects of care. It includes a whole section on continence and bladder and bowel care, giving the components that need to be in place for effective continence management and to implement measures to improve quality, which in turn will contribute to the introduction of clinical governance at local level. The Essence of Care Benchmarking Tool has provided a means of evaluating and comparing services, measuring current levels of performance and setting levels of best practice. This has been widely used and has been demonstrated to improve services to the patient where it has been utilised.

In 2006 the Department of Health published *Our Health, Our Care, Our Say: a new direction for community services*. This has probably had a significant impact on the provision of continence services, which are predominantly community-based. The aim of this policy is to reform health and social care through 'a radical and sustained shift in the way in which services are delivered . . . gives people a stronger voice so that they are the main drivers of service improvement'. One of the persistent problems of community care has been the poor coordination between health and local authorities. Historically, there have been incentives to move the costs onto others and disputes about who should provide care. Efforts to promote joint working were made but the fragmentation of health and social services remain a serious problem. The Government's rationale for this current shift is that people want more convenience, better access and more local coordination between services, described in the White Paper as 'more choice and a louder voice'. Tackling inequalities in health is also a key driver that focuses on both local need and vulnerable groups. A further driver is technological change, which allows patients to be treated more locally outside of the acute services, utilising, for example, telemedicine.

There is also a goal for more care to be undertaken outside hospital and in the home, with a huge drive to create fairness in accessing GP services (Cartmail, 2006). The other achievement sought is to invest in preventative care to avoid future costs. This ranges from broad public health measures to better care for people with long-term conditions and disabilities, which are sure to be affected by continence issues.

The National Director for Primary Care (Department of Health, 2007) states that the abiding message of *Our Health, Our Care, Our*

Say concerns the need to coordinate services. Patients, community nurses, pharmacists, voluntary organisations – even social enterprises and the private sector – should strive to work more closely together in order to provide better services and better outcomes for patients.

Nursing role

Nurses are accountable to the Nursing and Midwifery Council (NMC), which has a professional code of conduct. The twenty-first century has witnessed a growing body of regulation concerning record-keeping and the role of the nurse has extended to include nurse prescribing and the introduction of nurse-led services, such as walk-in centres (WICs), and autonomous roles such as nurse consultant and community matron. This section details changes to the traditional role of the nurse and looks at implications for continence care.

Community nurses are employed by Primary Care Trusts working alongside other members of the primary health care team and are usually responsible for undertaking continence care in the community setting.

From their beginnings as *public health nurses*, the primary role of community nurses has always been to look after the sick rather than to promote health. Although there have been various initiatives, such as community support teams, these have also been to look after the sick at home, thus reducing hospital admissions rather than promoting health. *Our Health, Our Care, Our Say* (Department of Health, 2007) aims to deliver better prevention services with earlier intervention, and to tackle health inequalities outside the hospital and in the home. However, this may not always be appropriate for solely the community nurse; more types of health care professional may become involved with the promotion of continence in primary care. Care pathways are ideal for this, as will become clear as we explore these later in the chapter.

The NHS Improvement Plan (2004) describes a new clinical role for nurses. Known as *community matrons*, these experienced, skilled nurses use case management techniques with patients who meet criteria denoting a very high-intensity use of health care. The case management work of community matrons is central to the Government's policy for the management of people with long-term conditions. The community matron will listen to the patient's views and design care around their needs, and ensure that that care is properly coordinated. It is anticipated that this will help prevent emergency admission to secondary care. Many patients with long-term conditions will suffer from continence problems and will benefit from this holistic approach to care.

One case history was of a patient with chronic obstructive pulmonary disease (COPD) who was a frequent attendee at the local Emergency Department and often requested home visits from his GP. He had been admitted to hospital five times in the last year. The community matron found out that when the patient took his diuretic tablets he could not get upstairs to the toilet in time so he just stopped taking the medication. The solution to the problem was simple and by the provision of aids to continence the hospital admissions reduced considerably, thereby saving the NHS money.

The Secretary of State for Health at the time said that she wanted to see 5% of the NHS budget (£4 billion) per year transferred from secondary care to primary care over the next ten years (Kmietowicz, 2006).

It has been suggested that many aspects of promoting health could carry on outside practice with lay trainers so that nursing professionals would have more time for patients with acute and chronic disease. With the potential shortage of nurses in the community it may be that aspects of care currently in the nursing domain will be commissioned from other sources.

Providers of care

The Labour Party's manifesto of 2005 committed the incoming Government to work with social enterprises as a stimulus to the third sector wherever possible. The third sector was to be promoted by the Department of Health as an alternative to public sector providers of health and social care services, and the resulting mix of models and sectors, combined with new commissioning priorities, was intended to help realign service provision across a range of organisations. This project was to track and influence the developing policy agenda (Royal College of Nursing, 2007). *Our Health, Our Care, Our Say* states, 'we will remove barriers to entry for the third sector as service providers for primary care' (Department of Health, 2006a).

Timmins (2006) makes the point that for-profit providers are ready to sweep into community and primary care, and that if too much time passes before social enterprises take shape then there may be little left for them. Timmins predicts that this will particularly apply to the new models of general practice, where it expects competition to be particularly fierce, and this could include all nurse-led services. It does admit, however, that there is relatively scant empirical evidence to demonstrate the tangible benefits of social enterprise in health care sectors.

It is proposed that the Primary Care Trusts become commissioning-only bodies and that community care will be wholly commissioned rather than directly provided. Strong commissioning of continence services will be vital, and high-quality commissioning will require strong and innovative leaders who understand the local community and workforce as well as the importance of clinical and organisational quality.

Care pathways can form the basis of standards to be met by the providers of care via the commissioning process. The Government, in its paper *The New NHS: Modern and Dependable* (Department of Health, 1997), states that the process of modernisation will replace the internal market with integrated care. Therefore, it is even more important to find a mechanism that will ensure equity of service provision at the front line in order to reduce variation in care. Care pathways can form the basis of the quality of care which patients should be able to expect from whosoever provides it.

It is not sufficient to state that the assessment should take place but to direct the tool with which to achieve it. Care pathways, because of the fact that they are intended to be dynamic, give immediate and valid access to audit data, which means that the quality of the care delivered is testable throughout the cycle.

Patient-centred care

In order to modernise and rebuild the health service the Government has produced some underpinning values that are known as *NHS core principles*. Ten core principles underpin *The NHS Plan* (Department of Health, 2000a), and they are designed to represent common ground between the Government's goals and what the NHS is capable of delivering. These core principles are the blocks for modernisation and reform that are needed to 'reshape the NHS from a patient's point of view' (Department of Health, 2000a).

The NHS Plan talks of the need for patients to be at the centre of care, for staff to focus on the patient's journey and to use evidence-based practice to provide care. Services will be shaped around the needs and preferences of individuals, which will mean health care professionals seeking to meet the various needs of different populations in an effort to improve the quality of service provision for all. *The NHS Plan* states that patients will receive planned programmes of care based on individual needs. Patients will no longer be recipients of care but will have a real say in the NHS, as 'we . . . transform the Health Service so that it is redesigned around the needs of patients', unlike in the past, when it was designed around budgets and tasks.

Background to continence care

The enormous cost of incontinence, as previously described, is an indication of how common the problem is. However, as previously stated, it was not until the 1970s that continence services started to develop. Prior to this no continence assessments were carried out. In the community, district nurses may have, during a general nursing assessment, included an enquiry about the patient's bladder or bowel function, but did not make any intervention. The outcome and the expectation of both nurse and patient was that there would be a supply of pads. These would be either disposable bed pads made of recycled pulp or a straight bulky disposable pad, which was held in place by plastic pants. For men there was a two-piece disposable device that was strapped onto the penis and was available from a hospital appliance fitter.

Urethral catheterisation was frequently used as a method of management. The catheters used were often of a large diameter and large balloon size, as this was thought to prevent leakage. Research has subsequently shown that it is the smallest catheters which actually prevent leakage. Catheterisation also has a high morbidity rate attached to it and causes considerable demands on services (Kohler-Ockmore and Feneley, 1996).

Continence care was often task-orientated rather than being built around the needs of the individual or their priorities, and no formal training on continence was available. Staff in some residential, nursing and long-stay homes would say that they toileted everyone every two hours, rather than recording how frequently the patient used the toilet, which would have established an individual regime that would have suited the patient.

Mobility was often made difficult or impossible for patients by the use of chairs that had fixed trays which did not allow the patient to get out of the chair. The use of open-backed gowns also discouraged independence.

In some areas the policy was not to use incontinence pads. This might have resulted in patients who required physiotherapy being returned from treatment because they had been incontinent. Likewise, not using fixation pants for pads meant that physiotherapy or mobilising was difficult.

In the early 1970s Dame Phyllis Friend, who was the Chief Nursing Officer at the Department of Health, wrote to district health authorities suggesting that they appoint a nursing officer to take responsibility for meeting the needs of people with incontinence (Chief Nursing Officer, 1977).

The nurses who initially became interested in incontinence were research nurses working in urodynamic units. They recognised the need to set up a multidisciplinary interest group, and this led to the formation of the Association of Continence Advisors (ACA) (now the Association for Continence Advice). In 1981 a nurse wrote to health authorities, seeking to identify interested professionals. This resulted in 100 people attending a meeting, demonstrating that there was, indeed, even then concerns about continence care.

A postal survey of urinary incontinence in the community carried out in 1980 had an amazingly high response rate of 89%. It showed a prevalence of 8.5% in females and 1.6% in males aged 15–64 and 11.6% in women and 6.9% in males aged 65 and over (Thomas *et al.*, 1980).

During the 1980s, many continence nurse specialists were appointed and services established and by the end of the decade there were 300 nurse specialists and two physiotherapists in specialist posts (Mandelstam, 1989). It should be noted that many continence nurse specialists were appointed to try to control the vastly overspent disposables budget. However, the quality of care for patients improved owing to:

■ the use of continence assessments
■ the provision of a quality service and evidence-based care

- professional input and advice
- continence education programmes
- the promotion of continence
- skilled services being available
- joint specialist clinics
- cost control
- male catheterisation by district nurses
- satellite clinics
- bladder scanning
- the advertisement of services
- improved appliances and equipment
- patient and staff information leaflets.

From the 1980s individual trusts had produced continence assessment forms. Many were not evidence-based, and nor had they been validated but were simply data-collection tools based on the experiences of the continence nurse specialist at the time.

The object of reducing spending on continence products resulted in assessment tools becoming the drivers for controlling costs rather than for the provision of high-quality care to the incontinent person (Bayliss et al., 2000). District nurses referred to the assessment as a pad assessment rather than an assessment of the person's status.

It was not until the 1990s that public awareness campaigns started to take place. In 1994 the first national public awareness campaign, 'Don't suffer in silence', was supported by leaflets, posters and toilet stickers. Since then each year has had a different theme. Events have been staged in town centres, railway stations, chemists, libraries, gyms and many other venues. Celebrities have been involved. All this has resulted in valuable media coverage. This has helped to change attitudes to incontinence and to encourage patients to seek help.

Information is now readily available on the Internet as continence organisations and manufacturers have easily accessible and helpful websites, giving both clinical advice and product information. Such information is provided in Chapter 8.

To facilitate better levels of continence care continence nurse specialists, physiotherapists and occupational therapists began providing in-house training on the promotion of continence and other related subjects. Now many Trusts make continence training for nurses mandatory. Short courses and modules on the promotion of continence and the management of incontinence are provided by universities throughout the United Kingdom, whilst the University of Ulster provides online training with the Foundation of Adult Urinary Incontinence (http://campusone.ulster.ac.uk/potential/shortcourses.php?cid=14).

The evolution of care pathways

Care pathways are known by many different names, some of which are:

- multidisciplinary pathways of care (MPCs)
- integrated care pathways (ICPs)
- anticipated recovery pathways (ARPs)
- clinical guidelines, or algorithms
- care maps
- critical paths.

ICPs used in health care have their origins in the United States of America, where the health care system is insurance-based. They were a means of standardising outcomes of patient care and controlling costs. Their introduction to the United Kingdom in the late 1980s was for a different reason: to achieve quality improvement. The first pathways were used in secondary care in planned surgery. This was because care was more easily predictable than in other sectors, and because some standardised practice was already in place. Since then their use has spread to almost every branch of health care, including continence care. The National Pathways Association has over 250 members representing secondary care, primary care, health trusts and the independent sector.

Structured multidisciplinary care plans identify essential steps in the patient health journey with the expected outcomes. These can be for a variety of conditions and procedures. ICPs have been in use since the 1980s but have become even more important with the introduction of legislation to raise the quality of care and standards across the NHS. An ICP is an anticipated plan of care for use by multidisciplinary teams which provides an appropriate timeframe in order to ensure that patients move through a condition or set of symptoms in order to experience a positive outcome (Middleton and Roberts, 2000). It specifies key events, tests, interventions and assessments occurring in a timely fashion to produce the best prescribed outcomes, within the resources and activities available for an appropriate episode of care (Wilson, 1996). In practice this describes, in advance, the care of patients within specific case types. The case type may be diagnostic, such as hip replacement, procedural, such as lumbar puncture, or conditional, such as pain.

Whatever the case type, there are common strands which are mapped out on the care pathway, which is then used as a clinical guideline, with the practitioner using their clinical judgement on whether to follow the anticipated care of the care pathway or to deviate from that care. Decisions to deviate from the care may be made for a variety of reasons, such as patient condition, lack of consent by the patient, lack of resources or the inappropriate skills of the caregiver. Such deviations are recorded as part of the care pathway's documentation, thus providing a facility by which care may be individualised as appropriate (Johnson, 1997). Such deviations are usually known as *variances*. It is these variances that make the difference between clinical guidelines, protocols and algorithms, none of which have the facility to actually record why the prescribed care was not given. Interventions may have much in common, but patients are different, and the skill of the caregiver comes from being able to differentiate between, and make clinical judgements about, various interventions and how appropriate they are for the individual patient. Care pathways allow clinical freedom, in a way that clinical protocols do not, whilst maintaining a high standard of care.

By using integrated care pathways to provide care for patients, staff are clear about the planned clinical care. The pathway will incorporate best evidence-based guidelines. It will provide a common record for all disciplines involved in the delivery of care. The patient outcomes are measured, and they allow variances to be tracked and performance to be reviewed (De Luc and Todd, 2003).

Benefits of care pathways

With the use of integrated care pathways it is clear that there are many benefits for both the patient and the organisation. Randomised controlled trials have been carried out by Sulch *et al.* (2002), and their findings state that 'integrated care pathways may improve assessment and communication, even in specialist . . . settings'. Teams can use integrated care pathways in order to plan the journey of the patient through the health care system. As maps are used for road travel, so integrated care pathways can be used for patients' journeys (Rees *et al.*, 2004). They found that, whilst members of the implementations teams were clear about the potential benefits, team leaders were resistant to the pathway because of a lack of resources and increased administration. The implementation therefore lacked clear leadership. Sulch *et al.* (2002) report that, even where no direct improvement in patient care arose from the introduction of pathways, there was a significant improvement in documentation and communications with both patients and GPs. Kent and Chalmers (2006) state that pathways are superior to traditional documentation when it comes to recording evidence of best practice. However, it would be speculation as to whether this reflects a direct improvement in delivery or an improvement in the quality of the documentation.

Putting the patient at the centre of the pathway is essential for it to be effective, and service users should be involved from the outset. Evidence has shown that pathways provide patients with a more realistic expectation of their treatment options and care progression (Middleton and Roberts, 2000). In their study Kent and Chalmers (2006) report that 60% of patients described that a pathway helped them understand their own care and helped in discussions with staff. Moreover, 68% reported a reduction in anxiety levels, and 82% thought that pathways were a better way of documenting their care.

It can be seen therefore that there are many drivers for the use of care pathways, from stronger commissioning of services, through equity, an audit trail and patient preference. Together with the Government initiatives outlined in *Our Health, Our Care, Our Say* (Department of Health, 2006a), which promotes the need for the patient to be at the centre of care and the probable changes in the way in which services should be provided, care pathways are a robust and effective tool for the treatment and management of all continence problems.

Key summary points

- Continence care is becoming more of a national priority.
- The role of the nurse is changing rapidly and more types of providers are involved in the provision of continence care.

- With the increase in providers care pathways ensure equity of care.
- Pathways demonstrate improvements in the provision of care to patients.
- Continence care has evolved into a real speciality with its own training agenda.
- Care pathways are standards which give the health care professional the clinical freedom to change care to suit the needs of the individual.
- Research shows patients prefer the care pathway approach.

Chapter 2

The impact of quality and the need for evidence

To demonstrate how severely patients can be affected this chapter begins with anecdotal evidence from patients about the impact of incontinence on their quality of life. It sets out both the case for change and the requirement to base health care practice on research in terms of improved patient outcomes. It goes on to describe an audit project by the authors which looks at how care to patients can be improved and gives the methodology for recording evidence and analysing the research to identify the good practice that was used in the development of the pathways. At the end of the chapter a case study is used to demonstrate a care pathway in action.

The patient's perspective

If I could walk again or get control of my bladder and bowels, I've no doubt which I'd choose: walking would be great, but the wheelchair doesn't stop me from doing things, the incontinence does. Did you know flight attendants can't help you to the toilet because it's against health and safety? So I can't travel long haul on my own. (Janet, aged 42)

Just going shopping is a major event. I know where all the loos are and I can't spend too long on anything. It would be lovely to try clothes on but I daren't. But really, what's the point? I can only buy stuff that covers up my pads anyway. (Fiona, aged 35)

My son wants me to visit but I can't: I won't travel and I'm terrified of wetting his bed. He doesn't know I've got this problem and I don't want him to. I can't carry all these pads and I wouldn't know where to put the used ones if I did. I'm not going. (George, aged 77)

I've leaked ever since my last baby and he's a father now. I thought it's part of being a woman. My mum had it, and my sister, so why should I be any different? I nearly didn't come when my doctor referred me but I was worried that if I didn't I might not get any more appointments. (Karen, aged 52)

Perhaps no other symptom causes quite so much emotion as incontinence. In discussion the patients often felt overwhelmed by the sheer effects of the problem as every part of their lives were affected by it. Few other conditions cause as much shame and embarrassment and affect quality of life to such an extent. Many sufferers do not seek help and are unaware that many things can be done to help them manage, improve or even cure their incontinence. Owing to people's reluctance to discuss their incontinence, many old wives' tales have grown up about the condition. For example, the common or garden weed the dandelion was known in the seventeenth century as *piss-a-bed* and it was believed that it caused incontinence. In modern French the plant is called *pissenlit*, which translates similarly and presumably for the same reasons. A brief review of the Internet suggests causes of cystitis as bicycle riding, wearing miniskirts and not sitting on toilet seats while urinating. (http://clinmed.netprints.org/cgi/content/full/2000050003v1). None of this has any evidence to support it.

Many women believe that it is natural, following childbirth, to leak when exercising. Indeed, as the symptom is so common, when they confide in a friend or relative they often find that their confidantes have the same problem, which encourages the belief that it is only to be expected. It has to be acknowledged that it is really only since towards the end of the last century that incontinence has been taken seriously as a speciality and that genuine high-quality research has taken place.

Evidence-based practice

The importance of quality, equity and standards is driven home throughout many Government White Papers, from *A First Class Service* (Department of Health, 1998) and *The Essence of Care*

(Department of Health, 2001), a patient-focused benchmarking kit that includes a section on continence, through to the *National Service Frameworks*, which set national standards and identify key interventions for a defined service or care group (e.g. Department of Health, 2001a). The Government describes them as forming one of a range of measures to raise quality and decrease variations in service, introduced in *The New NHS* (Department of Health, 1997) and *A First Class Service* (Department of Health, 1998). *The NHS Plan* re-emphasized the role of *National Service Frameworks* as drivers in delivering the modernisation agenda (Department of Health, 2000a).

Evidence-based practice is well articulated in the body of literature of which the following are examples.

Evidence based medicine is the conscientious, explicit, and judicious use of current best evidence in making decisions about the care of individual patients. The practice of evidence based medicine means integrating individual clinical expertise with the best available external clinical evidence from systematic research. By individual clinical expertise we mean the proficiency and judgement that individual clinicians acquire through clinical experience and clinical practice. Increased expertise is reflected in many ways, but especially in more effective and efficient diagnosis and in the more thoughtful identification and compassionate use of individual patients' predicaments, rights, and preferences in making clinical decisions about their care. By best available external clinical evidence we mean clinically relevant research, often from the basic sciences of medicine, but especially from patient centred clinical research into the accuracy and precision of diagnostic tests (including the clinical examination), the power of prognostic markers, and the efficacy and safety of therapeutic, rehabilitative, and preventive regimens. External clinical evidence both invalidates previously accepted diagnostic tests and treatments and replaces them with new ones that are more powerful, more accurate, more efficacious, and safer. (Sackett et al., 1996)

Evidence-based practice (EBP) is an approach to health care wherein health professionals use the best evidence possible, i.e. the most appropriate information available, to make clinical decisions for individual patients. EBP values, enhances and builds on clinical expertise, knowledge of disease mechanisms, and pathophysiology. It involves complex and conscientious decision-making based not only on the available evidence but also on patient characteristics, situations, and preferences. It recognizes that health care is individualized and ever changing and involves uncertainties and probabilities. Ultimately EBP is the formalization of the care process that the best clinicians have practiced for generations. (McKibbon, 1998)

The case for change

However devoted and dedicated to evidence-based care, continence budgets are competing with many others, many of which are of a higher priority, and so cost controls have to be applied. This has caused an overload on continence services, some of which have waiting lists to receive products (Dolman, 1998), and have to deal with the cost versus quality-of-life dilemma. The edges of quality of continence care and budgetary control have become blurred as many continence services institute a 'no pads without a continence assessment form' policy.

However, health care professionals have many demands on their time. The drive to keep people in their own homes with increasing levels of dependency in the community means that a community nurse must prioritise his/her caseload, and so a continence assessment has low priority against, for example, meeting the needs of a patient who may otherwise be admitted to secondary care. To facilitate better levels of continence care, continence services provide ongoing training and education. However, in practice the same interested nurses attend the education sessions, so the interest and motivation of the health care professionals who see the patient determine the quality of the service provided. Patients who remain incontinent have a poorer quality of life and are a continual drain on health service resources.

For many years, there has been pressure to reduce spending on continence products. However, from almost no assessment at all, this has resulted in assessment tools being used to control costs instead of providing high-quality care for the incontinent person. The authors involved in this project found, for their own Trusts, that still when continence assessment takes place by health care professionals it is with the aim of providing a pad. Indeed, it is not uncommon for the assessment to be referred to as a *pad assessment* rather than as a *continence assessment*. This is rather like referring to a *wound assessment* as a *dressing assessment*.

Assessment forms may be submitted to the continence service for checking, for quality issues, and because of the need for cost containment. For example, some policies state that no more that three pads per 24-hour period may be supplied. This checking of the assessment forms can cause conflict between continence services and the Health care professional, to the detriment of the patient.

So, are assessment forms a satisfactory method of providing good continence care?

Audit project

The first step in the process was to check whether assessment forms as a data-collection tool were providing continence advice and support. To this end, a baseline audit was undertaken of 300 patients, described in detail in Bayliss *et al.* (2000). A postal questionnaire was sent to randomly selected community patients who had recently (within the last six months) been assessed by a community nurse. Continence nurse specialists involved in the audit had over a period of time undertaken regular education and training sessions with the community staff concerned. However, for the purposes of eliminating bias, the audit was carried out independently. Ninety-seven per cent of the sample patients had their assessment carried out by a district nurse. Eighty-three per cent were female and 90% were over the age of 60. Although urine testing should have formed part of the assessment, only 4% had been requested to provide a sample at their initial assessment. Patients were asked a series of questions, concerning:

- what advice they had been given
- what tests they had received
- what the long-term view of their prognosis was
- levels of incontinence.

A high response rate was not anticipated as it was felt that patients would be too embarrassed to complete the questionnaires, despite anonymity. A response rate of 30–40% is usually expected from postal questionnaires (McNeill, 1990). However, despite low expectations, the response rate was 67%, giving the first lesson: incontinent patients want to be involved in their care. Many of the questionnaires were written in detail, demonstrating that patients wanted to share their feelings and perceptions. It is interesting to note that the majority of the comments were concerned with aspects of treatment and not the provision or quality of products, despite being in receipt of products from the NHS.

Contemporaneously with the questionnaire, and to further inform the process, an audit was made of the assessment forms relating to the same patients and checked to see how closely the information provided by health care professionals and the patients' understanding matched. The purpose of this was to study the care that patients actually perceived that they had received. For example, many health care professionals had stated that they had taught pelvic floor exercises, but patients reported that they did not remember them. This did not demonstrate that patients had not been taught pelvic floor exercises but that they did not remember them, and illustrates a need for better patient information.

The audit results reinforced the belief that patients did not receive either an equitable service or appropriate information. The majority of patients were motivated enough to complete the questionnaire, and many stated that they wished to improve their continence status. It is not suggested that any patient's continence status worsened as a result of nursing intervention, but that more in the status quo category could have improved. Only 20% showed some improvement, a figure markedly below that given by the Royal College of Physicians of 70% to 80% (Royal College of Physicians, 1995). There was indeed evidence to show that delivery of continence care in the community could be improved.

The care pathway solution

The solution that seemed to meet all the objectives was the care pathway process. Pathways anticipate and describe in advance, by the use of evidence, the care of patients within specific case types. Moreover, the process is dynamic, and regular monitoring and review change the pathway as advances are made and variances are identified. The pathway provides the appropriate intervention(s) whilst allowing clinical freedom through the variance tracking process.

The evidence

The contents of the pathways in terms of the clinical standards and the organisation, sequence and method are based on the evidence, as set out in the literature on continence care.

The literature review took the form of a search of the databases CINAHL, Medline and NHS Net, which produced over 2000 items.

It was first written up in a series of three articles about pathways for continence care (Bayliss *et al.*, 2000a). Exclusions then included veterinary articles and non-translated foreign language papers. It was also decided to limit search of the literature to the previous five years only. The review produced 400 articles, documents, books and other sources to investigate and read. A computerised database, Microsoft Access, was used to store records and for easy access.

Each entry on the database had details about the author, article and an abstract. Also, the data were categorised into evidence types: RCT (randomised control trial), non-RCT, case controlled or case matched studies, cohort and longitudinal studies, case studies, reviews, guidelines, evaluations and discussion/description. This followed the orthodox hierarchy of evidence, with RCTs as the gold standard (see, for example, http://www.shef.ac.uk/scharr/ir/units/systrev/hierarchy.htm).

The purpose of categorising the data was to determine the strength of evidence on a particular standard or method relevant to continence care. The evidence was not always clear-cut, as RCTs sometimes contradicted one another.

To ensure the accurate and legitimate application of the evidence the category of evidence was not the only indicator used. As important is the validity of the research, that is how far the research reflects the true nature of the subject that is being researched; for example, if bladder training is shown to work in an inpatient setting, will this be equally valid should the patient be in the community or are there other variable factors which need to be taken into account? The quantity of the data was used to validate the quality. Therefore, where two evaluation articles were in agreement about an intervention, this was deemed stronger than one RCT.

The evidence was then further categorised into keywords. The authors had decided that three pathways would initially be designed, for stress incontinence, urge incontinence and overflow incontinence. Therefore, all data, which had reference to these types of incontinence, were grouped as such within the database.

The data needed to be arranged so that it would be possible to search within each item. Eight further keywords were used, including *quality of life, compliance, audit, evidence base* and *cognitive dysfunction*. This allowed searches to take place that would accurately inform each item on the care pathway. For instance, for the stress incontinence pathway all the articles that related to the keywords *pelvic floor* could be quickly identified. The actual data were kept

Table 2.1 Search data

Category of research	Keywords (1)	Type	Keywords (2)
RCT, NRCT			Pelvic floor
Case controlled study		Assessment/ screening	Older patient
Reviews	Stress		Cognitive dysfunction
Cohort/longitudinal study	Urge	Treatment/ intervention	Compliance
Surveys			Neurological
Evaluations	Overflow		Voiding dysfunction
Guidelines		Audit/ outcome	Primary care
Audit			Medication
Discussion/ description	Mixed		Quality of life

numerically in files, allowing for easy access. Moreover, it was possible to search under three further headings, which could be needed in any pathway: *assessment/screening*, *treatment/intervention* and *audit/outcome*. Searches could be extremely specific or much more general.

Table 2.1 demonstrates how searches may be made. Once the search had taken place, the computer would give the numbers of the articles which were specific to the search.

Other sources of evidence

Other sources were identified and visits took place. Particularly useful was the Dynamic Quality Improvement Programme of the Royal College of Nursing, which had produced the *Directory of NHS Trusts Using Care Pathways* (Royal College of Nursing Institute, 1998) and provided much help and guidance on care pathways and their application. The National Pathways Association and Continence Foundation also contributed valuable material. Lines of enquiry had to be followed if only to discover what was not being undertaken.

It is not suggested that such detailed examination of the literature is necessary for the purposes of the adoption of these pathways. However, it must always be borne in mind that new research is constantly published and, in order that the pathways are dynamic, must be incorporated into reviews. The authors have continued to review the literature and to keep the database up to date, adding relevant references to the database and incorporating appropriate modifications to the pathways.

Outcome of evidence base and variance tracking

The usefulness of the evidence must be constantly analysed. The pathways must be constantly updated to reflect the needs of the target population, as well as new research. A system is necessary to ensure that this happens, as without this they are not care pathways but merely protocols, frozen in the time in which they were designed.

Care pathways create the opportunity to track the reasons why a professional has been unable or unwilling to carry out a prescribed action. They provide the means to state the circumstances and give a reason. This can be as simple as an extra line on the paperwork or may be part of a computerised patient record. This system is known as *variance tracking* (Kitchiner, 1997). Such variances from the expected care will form the basis for investigation on whether the pathway should be amended to take into account the issues surrounding the variation. For instance, when the pathways were originally designed an assumption was made that all staff had access to urine testing equipment and that it would be of the same type. Therefore, a space for entry of data was inserted into the pathway so that the results could be recorded. On the first (six-monthly) variance track it was discovered that some community nurses did not have access to dipsticks and therefore sent specimens of urine to the pathology laboratory if they felt that the patient had symptoms of a urinary infection. Others were borrowing dipsticks from the practice nurses, who had a different type that did not include nitrite and leucocyte test pads, which were the factors used to identify whether or not the patients had a urinary infection. Clearly, this did not give patients an equitable service. The nurses had been told that they could not have dipsticks, because they go out of date so quickly. A solution was found by having a central supply where the nurses could access smaller amounts, and all patients thereafter had their urine routinely dip tested – a recommendation from the evidence base.

As more evidence about caffeine has been identified, caffeine fading has been added into the pathway. Initially, patients were being told to stop drinking caffeinated drinks if they had any degree of voiding urgency. However, the compliance with this was very poor as they would almost certainly get a significant withdrawal headache and go back to drinking caffeine. Research has shown that caffeine fading is much more tolerable and therefore has better compliance (Juliano and Griffiths, 2004). This was incorporated into the amendments, with much better outcomes.

It can be seen clearly that pathways must be reviewed regularly to be truly effective.

Next steps

Once you have the evidence, the next step is to process map. This process involves mapping out the patient's journey as they come into contact with continence services. This helps service providers appreciate any key issues and frustrations for the patient and the map becomes a source of reference for the development and implementation of pathways.

To return to the patients quoted at the beginning of the chapter, intervention by continence nurse specialists made a significant difference to each one. Janet had multiple sclerosis and is a fiercely independent lady who wanted to travel before she became too frail. A change in management methods allowed her to travel long haul and maintain her dignity and privacy. Fiona had taken to self-help for her symptoms, cutting down radically on her fluid intake and passing urine far too frequently. Some judicious advice and a change of medication meant a substantial change in her quality of life. George could not be persuaded to tell his son about his condition or to use a different product and is continuing to receive support in the hope he changes his mind. Karen is perhaps the greatest success story, having undertaken a course of physiotherapy she is now dry, has lost three stone in weight and her self-esteem is very high. It can be seen therefore that small interventions after careful assessment can make a great difference. So how do we go about change?

A case study of the adoption of continence care pathways

A clinical nurse specialist in continence care decided to implement care pathways in her area shortly after they were first published in 2000. In 2008 she was interviewed to look at the effect that this implementation had on the care provided for that area.

Why did you implement care pathways? Was it part of a process mapping exercise or service redesign?

Care pathways were implemented as part of a process of redesign. It was clear that assessment forms were inefficient in collecting the right sort of information required to make a diagnosis and facilitate onward treatment. Generally, health care professionals either did not complete or inadequately completed the forms and did not understand why they were required to ask the questions. Despite education they were not able to form an accurate diagnosis and therefore collecting the data was both a waste of time and unhelpful for the patient. Care pathways were a way of introducing a logical tool, which could be used without too much training or resources. A questionnaire was sent out to ascertain what health care professionals thought of and wanted from the paperwork, which they had to complete. They were asked how it influenced outcomes for patients and what they would like to have as a tool. Generally, the consensus was that health care professionals wanted shorter, easier-to-use and more effective assessment forms.

Process mapping did not take place, as this was not recommended at the time. However, it is easy to see how valuable the process mapping system is and we would definitely undertake this process if introducing further pathways.

What difficulties did you have in implementation? What were you expecting by introducing care pathways?

Health care professionals did take them on board in essence. Although they could see the benefits, not everyone tested urine or promoted the use of the urinary journals. They gave their reasons as not having enough time, but there is also a strong suspicion that despite the fact that they did not like the previous data-collection tool they also did not like change.

The expectation was that higher-quality assessments would take place, ensuring that all patients would have had a better assessment, during which patients would be treated for symptoms rather than just given products, or although they may be supplied with products they were also treated. There is a theory that more efficient assessments will save money, because more people being treated means that fewer products are provided. Although this seems logical, the increase in treatment generally coincides with an increase in referral levels as more people have their quality of life improved and spread the word.

It is the experience of this area that when the continence service is easily accessible and supports the staff the health care professionals using the care pathways are more confident and understand the need for the pathways, which in turn makes them more effective. If the support system slips, then so does the quality of the assessment.

Did you involve patients and carers in the introduction?

We have a user support group which comprised people who had expressed an interest in championing the service, patients who were currently in receipt of products from the service, a representative of the private sector for nursing and residential care, and patients who have had continence problems and have been assessed and feel able to talk about the outcome. There was also some professional input from occupational therapists and physiotherapists. They meet every two months for discussion and feedback, and this group was consulted on the pathways and its views were incorporated. Again, in retrospect it would have been better to consult with a much wider group of users in order that their needs could be met.

How did you localise them?

User group meetings and professional meeting forums were set up to look at whether the entire pathway applied to the local service. In fact, changes were minimal and mainly around the need to include local administration numbers to input onto the computer system in order to identify patients for audit purposes. After the first audit a back sheet was also added to request information about patients' previous medical histories, particularly their obstetric history and to identify whether there was anything else that the patients felt was relevant. It was felt that if the health care professional undertaking the assessment was interested in looking at the patient's symptoms in more depth and therefore diagnosing and treating the patient the back sheet would assist with this. This may be part of the process of letting go of the old assessment tool. The information did not add to the direct care on the care pathway, but it did satisfy the needs of some of the staff who wanted to gain the information. The sheet was not compulsory for completion, but an addendum. Even within the continence team there was resistance to change. A few members of staff sought to bypass the specific pathways because, first and foremost, they represented a great deal of paperwork.

What benefits have you seen?

Assessments are more thorough. More urine tested means that more infections are being treated. More constipation is being identified and treated and there is a higher awareness of the impact that some medications have on continence. One of the main benefits is that it is easy to audit and changes can be made and reviewed without resorting to other paperwork; all the information is there in the pathway.

Do you think care is now more equitable?

The level of care is still somewhat dependent on the interest of the nurse. Some basic elements are more equitable, certainly, as regards urine testing, constipation, environment and medication, but it is still a little patchy and dependent on the care provider to a degree. The experience here is that it needs time to get people to understand the essence of the care pathway, and new members of staff may not like or understand it if they are not used to using care pathways. It was thought that it would not be necessary to provide support, as pathways are independent and stand alone, but it has been found that when support is provided the compliance with using the pathways is much improved. For a health care professional, it can be quite daunting to be asked to believe that a certain action is the right evidence-based one to take, and they need the confidence in the system to be able to use the pathways independently. It might be that were pathways to be implemented local guidelines or protocols could be used to underwrite them, which would give more confidence in their use.

There is still a perception in some people's minds (health care professionals' as well as patients') that incontinence equals pads. Recently, there have been more television advertisements for pads, which rather reinforces that this is the way to treat continence problems. Unfortunately, the care pathway cannot change perceptions that nothing can be done and that pads are the only solution.

Are referrals more appropriate?

Referrals are definitely more appropriate. There are far fewer referrals for patients who have urinary tract infection or constipation, two big causes of incontinence, as they are screened out by the pathways before they ever get to the continence service.

The great advantage for the patient is that it reduces the patient journey. It is interesting to note, however, that the continence service also gets more referrals by health care professionals who are more aware of what can be achieved, because they get feedback from the care pathways. This increased awareness does help, and when a pathway has brought about an improvement that particular professional is happy to use it again.

Have you audited variances?

The variances have been audited and the pathways have been amended in the light of the results. For example, the pathway was amended so that patients could be more easily referred into the system at the end of the pathway. It was also identified that health care professionals needed more support at that point, and so a strategy was devised for this. However, it has to be admitted that variance tracking audit has not been carried out in the last two years because of time constraints. When the pathways were implemented, it was considered that the variance tracking could be undertaken on a regular, rolling basis. However, it is strongly recommended that a proper programme be put in place at the outset of implementation, as it is very easy to not undertake the audit when time constraints and other pressures are placed upon the service. The variance tracking is recognised as the most important part of the process. New users must have a variance tracking plan in place as part of care pathway implementation and should identify the necessary resources to support that plan.

The next chapter sets out in detail how the reader may wish to take this forward.

Key summary points

- Patients' quality of life is severely affected by incontinence.
- Practice requires an evidence base.
- A care pathway is a tool that enables practitioners to use an evidence base.
- Continence care should be about treatment, not cost containment.
- Audit showed that patients received neither an equitable service nor appropriate information.
- Variance tracking is an essential component of care pathways.
- Care pathways must be reviewed regularly to be effective.

Chapter 3

Process of development of care pathways

This chapter describes two ways in which continence care pathways can be developed. The first way of developing pathways is process mapping and service, or part service, redesign, and the second way adapts existing templates of pathways to fit local circumstances. These two methods are not mutually exclusive or necessarily alternatives to one another as process mapping not only can produce original pathways but also can provide for the local adoption of pathways. Which method used will depend on what is available in the way of time and resources as process mapping can be done locally so that local needs are met, or national pathways can be used.

One of the major challenges to the adoption of pathways is the resistance to change and so this chapter gives some ideas as to how the barriers may be overcome, including a significant section on techniques to improve communication with patients.

Advantages of care pathways

As stated in Chapter 2, the key arguments for the use of pathways are as follows:

- They are evidence-based, which makes them up to date and based on current good practice in continence care.
- They can be audited through variance tracking.
- They ensure consistency of care across providers.

- They lay out the patient assessment and clearly define the role of all the caregivers, and so minimise risk.
- They are developed with the patient being at the centre and involved, which results in better care and outcomes.

The benefits of care pathways are further detailed elsewhere in the literature (see, for example, De Luc and Todd (2003), Jones and Coyne (2001) and Johnson (1997)).

Process mapping and service redesign

Good practice now requires the creation of models of service improvement. These may be used to form the basis of care pathways rather than the existing structure of care provision, and help service providers appreciate any key issues and frustrations for the patient, and so the map becomes a source of reference for the development and implementation of pathways. To help draw the map and understand the patient's perspective it may be necessary to bring relevant staff and providers together at a specific event to discuss the current care provision.

The first step in process mapping is to identify the patient's journey and identify the points of contact with health services/professionals as the patient travels through the NHS. An example of a patient's journey involving a continence service may look a bit like this:

1. Doctor tells patient they need flow tests and doctor writes to continence service to request appointment.
2. Doctor tells patient appointment will come in the post.
3. Patient goes home to wait.
4. Patient receives appointment letter.
5. Patient goes to clinic.
6. Receptionist receives patient and checks details.
7. Patient seen by nurse specialist and tests undertaken.
8. Results are sent back to GP.
9. Patient waits at home.
10. Patient visits GP and receives results.

It is useful to break down processes into component parts like this as it allows one to see how the service comes together, and it is an exercise that the authors have conducted before, and one which is explored further in Chapter 4, in relation to mobility and cognitive function.

The process map of the patient's journey then needs analysis. To help with this process the following questions are posed in the *Improvement leaders' guide* (http://www.institute.nhs.uk/improvementleadersguides) *Process Mapping, Analysis and Redesign*:

- How many steps are there for the patient?
- How many times is the patient passed from one person to another (hand-off)?
- What is the approximate time taken for each step (task time)?
- What is the approximate time between each step (wait time)?
- What is the approximate time between the first and the last step?
- When does the patient join a queue or when is the patient put on a waiting list?
- Do these delays occur on a regular basis?
- How many steps add no value for the patient? Imagine that you, or your parent or child, is the patient. What steps add nothing to the care being received?
- Where are the problems for patients? What do patients complain about?
- Where are there problems for staff? (NHS Institute for Innovation and Improvement, 2005a).

The journey of the patient referred to the continence service for flow tests involves ten steps, and the patient may be passed from one person to another five times. There are not any target times for times taken for each step or between each step or between the first and the last step but the patient joins the queue for a diagnostic appointment or any subsequent treatment when the continence service gets the referral letter from the GP. Many of the steps add no value for the patient, like waiting for flow test appointments, which can take seven to eight weeks.

The *Choose and Book* scheme is intended to give patients more choice, giving the choice as to where and when they can go for their specialist care, including continence care. Under the Choose and Book scheme since 1 January 2006, patients requiring a first outpatient appointment are offered a choice of at least four hospitals or clinics, including an independent provider in some cases. Patients are also offered a choice as to the date and time of their first outpatient appointment. Currently, 25% of GP referrals to hospitals and clinics are now managed through the Choose and Book electronic system (http://www.chooseandbook.nhs.uk).

One of the problems that arise in the patient's journey is that they will often want to know what the results of any tests are at the clinic appointment. So, continuing with the flow test example, when the test is done, the patient will often want to know the results, perhaps understandably, rather than have to wait to hear from their GP. This is the *parallel process* referred to in the *Improvement leaders' guides* (NHS Institute for Innovation and Improvement, 2005), which suggests that certain processes, usually administrative, must be considered for review in order to avoid delaying patients or frustrating staff.

The reason the patient does not receive the results of the flow test at this stage is that it is not up to the continence service to say what is to happen but up to the GP, as the patient is a GP referral. Managing the patient's expectations as to what the continence service can offer is an issue and can depend on what information the patient has received from a GP as to their diagnosis of the their condition. In an attempt to manage patient expectations, one continence service sends out information to help patients understand why they are coming to see the continence service, an information sheet that was made up from frequently asked questions by patients. Points include:

- length of appointment and waiting time
- directions for bringing a urine specimen
- explanation of questionnaires enclosed with appointment
- possible outcomes.

It was noted that after these information sheets had been provided the 'did not attend' rate dropped significantly and the fact that patients understood why they were being asked to complete such paperwork meant that they were attending with the paperwork completed.

On the basis of the map, analysis and consideration of parallel processes, the next step is to redesign the patient's journey. This may involve the following elements:

- Coordinate the patient's progression through care
- Plan and schedule care at times to suit the patient

- Reduce the number of times a patient has to travel to visit the hospital or surgery.
- Reduce or eliminate batching.
- Reduce the number of queues to be managed.
- Extend staff roles (NHS Institute for Innovation and Improvement, 2005a).

So a redesigned patient journey involving flow testing may set up clinic sessions using the equipment at local GP surgeries, thereby decentralising the service. An alternative suggestion would be for the central clinic to lend out the equipment to GP surgeries whilst it was not being used by the continence service. It may be that a practice nurse could be trained to undertake the studies. This would then reduce travelling time for the patients and results could be given at the time of the scan with the GP there to say what is going to happen next on the basis of the patient's results.

The impact of any redesign of the patient's journey would then need to be evaluated using the PDSA (plan, do, study and act) cycle to test a change idea.

- **Plan:** agree the change to be tested or implemented.
- **Do:** carry out the test or change and measure the impact.
- **Study:** study data before and after the change and reflect on what was learnt.
- **Act:** plan the next change cycle or plan implementation (NHS Institute for Innovation and Improvement, 2005).

Change may be better or more easily implemented or accepted by those staff involved by making and evaluating one change at a time, for example introducing the bladder scanner to one GP practice at a time.

'Using the Plan, Do, Study, Act cycle has been like a breath of fresh air. I have found that it is much easier to convince staff to try out the change in a small way and then reflect on it and refine it as needed. They felt much more involved and therefore feel some ownership of the new process and I have found that this improves sustainability because the staff have themselves invested in it and agreed the change', quotation from a project manager from the south of England, in the *Improvement leaders' guides* (NHS Institute for Innovation and Improvement, 2005).

Local adaptation of template pathways

The evidence as described by the body of literature is the major starting point for writing the pathways. However, it is equally important to look at the local needs, requirements and available resources to ensure that an equitable and high-quality service will be supplied. The pathways will stand or fall by good application of local issues. Using an example of bladder scanning, the research is clear that post-void residual urine should be identified. However, this requires the use of ultrasound bladder scanners, which may not be available to all staff at all times. Therefore, it may be that a post-void catheterisation will have to be performed instead. If it is not clear in the pathway, then staff may just put a variance in, stating that a scanner was not available, instead of undertaking the alterative diagnostic test. These can be identified in a variety of ways.

Interviews

It is necessary to talk to all the key stakeholders who will be using or have an influence on the pathways. This can be done through group meetings or individual interviews. As the gold standard will be a pathway that follows the patient through primary and secondary care, each profession that will have an input into the pathway should be able to give their view. The evidence may state that mobility issues should be considered, but how, where, by whom and in what timeframe is a matter for local debate. The process mapping exercise should have taken this into account, but it is important to ensure that all stakeholders are on board with the action or intervention to be carried out or the variances will not be completed.

Pilots

Test a few pathways with an entry point, requesting detailed variances to see if there are any issues that have not been identified. Even just a few can identify gaps. It is perfectly acceptable, and indeed helpful, to attach a sheet of paper asking users how they felt about the actions they were asked to take and whether they encountered any difficulties in undertaking them.

Evaluation

Once the pilots have been evaluated and changed, then a formal Version 1 can be used. It is imperative that this is clearly marked with the date and version number as pathways must be dynamic and regularly updated. Sometimes, the updates may only be minor, and although old versions should be destroyed, only clear marking can identify which is which. As well as variances being incorporated at each evaluation, new research and changes in local resources should be investigated and acted upon.

Care Pathways can be seen as 'recipe book' medicine, and the criticism is made that 'one size fits all'. Each patient is different but the basic care provided should be equitable for all. It is the reverse of the postcode lottery, where all patients have equal and qualitative assessment. One of the major challenges to the adoption of pathways is the resistance to change, and so the next section of this chapter gives some ideas as to how this may be minimised through the use of communication skills.

Overcoming resistance to change

Bringing people together and ensuring that everyone is involved will mean that everyone feels ownership of change and therefore is less resistant to it. It may be felt that a meeting of all interested parties will not fundamentally change the outcome of the pathway and this may well be true. However, the success of the pathway will ride on people being prepared to use it properly, and they are far more likely to do this if they feel involved as part of the process: shareholders in the pathway. The driver for change here is an improvement in service delivery for the patient, and this focus must never be lost in the design and implementation stages.

Clear communication is paramount and the process must be transparent. The most effective use of pathways is not directive but achieved through consensus. The pathways will constantly be updated and changes can be made as a result of the variance tracking process, so pathways may always be viewed as a pilot that everyone can have an input into. The success of care pathways, as with all other assessment data, depends on the way they are used in practice.

Beliefs and values are the rules we live by, based on our own experience, and can act as self-fulfilling prophecies. Many patients define themselves by their beliefs around their condition, which influences their quality of life. This can lead to misconceptions and difficulties when lifestyle changes are discussed. For example, a patient who believes they are incontinent because they are getting old or because their mother was will resist change because they do not believe change will occur.

The effective use of pathways also involves understanding the patient's perception of their symptoms. Keeping a journal or diary of the symptoms can establish the problem or problems, demonstrate improvements and help the patient identify what they can do for themselves. Recommending lifestyle changes requires a change in behaviour by the patient. The pathway, by its very nature, highlights areas of change, which the health care professional is required to discuss with the patient. For example, recommending an increase or decrease of fluid intake or type of fluid, or dietary advice, can often be a challenge, and the patient's perception can increase their resistance to change. Without suitable and relevant information to take away and study, and the support of others to address this, success can be limited.

If you have the tools, you can do so much more for yourself. (Martha, aged 70, practising pelvic floor exercises and bladder retraining)

Improving communication with patients

The information gathered by the health care professional from the patient relies on the use of excellent communication skills. Using appropriate language will help the health care professional build a rapport with patients, who are expected to share sensitive and highly personal information in a short space of time. Patients want to feel that they have been listened to and that their concerns and fears have been heard (Henwood and Lister, 2007). It is clear that effective listening takes effort and concentration and is a learnt skill. Individuals should be listened to without judgement, distortion or analysis (O'Connor and Lages, 2004).

One distinctive element in providing a history of past illness relates to the difficulty patients may have in recalling accurately long-term, personal information. The accuracy of the answers may require a great deal of deep thought and the consequent time required for this. Generally, people are better at remembering events and actions rather than thoughts and intensities and therefore it may be helpful to try to correlate symptoms with life events and milestones. Further, the literature states that doctors tend to attend to the first issue mentioned by their patients, yet this is commonly not the issue which concerns them most (Gask and Usherwood, 2002), and recommends that the patient is allowed to finish talking and that open-ended questions and repetition are employed to check that the patient and assessor agree on the issues. Indeed, in one study Starfield *et al.* (1981) state that in 50% of consultations the patient and assessor did not agree on the nature of the main presenting problem. Listening, understanding and prioritisation are put forward as the keys to good outcomes. However, Lesser *et al.* (2005) warn of the danger of patients presenting opinion as fact or causally connecting events which are unrelated, which leads to a misconstruction of diagnosis. This demonstrates the value of paraphrasing and summarising the information provided by the patient. It is also important to be aware of patients' cues, indicating something they wish to talk about. A cue may be verbal, through hinting at other issues, or non-verbal, such as changing posture, eye contact or tone of voice (Gask and Usherwood, 2002).

There is no doubt that better communication improves outcomes but also that patient satisfaction with the interview strongly predicts compliance with treatment on both theoretical and empirical grounds (Little *et al.*, 2001). Moreover, they were able to demonstrate that symptom burden at one month was worse if expectations of a positive approach were not met. It is therefore imperative that a patient-centred approach is taken, in both time and in an environment that is conducive to the disclosure of information which the patient may find embarrassing. Patients who feel that they have not been treated well in communication terms feel that the consultation has been geared to the health professional's agenda, with enforcement of the medical model taking no account of the impact on the patient in anything other than physical terms. Patient-centred care demands a fusion of professional expertise on the part of the clinician and the experiential expertise of the patient (Dunn, 2003).

It must be emphasised that language is a key part of communication skills and that even if people speak the same language they will not all use the same descriptor for a given sensation. The effectiveness of verbal communication relies on both parties listening, hearing and assimilating the correct message (Roberts and Bucksey, 2007).

Shatell and Hogan (2005) assert that understanding can be facilitated by one overarching communication principle: nurses may not comprehend what patients mean. They go on to state that patients experience greater satisfaction when they feel that they have been truly understood.

It is important when paying attention to the patient to understand the importance of body language and how this will help create rapport with another person in a short space of time. Paying attention, mirroring and matching, whether the patient is sitting or standing, their posture, what words they use, their energy levels and being able to put yourself in the patient's shoes (for example considering how they are feeling about their symptoms) will improve the patient's experience and help the professional obtain the information they need more quickly to be able to treat or manage the patient more effectively. Improving the outcome for the health care professional as well as the patient encourages the use of the pathway.

Rapport can be described as communication, which creates trust, respect and recognition. When you are in rapport with another person, you will find that you match body language, tonality and gestures. Only about 7% of communication depends on the words we speak; body language and tonality make up the rest (Henwood and Lister, 2007). Body language reflects attitudes and feelings you have towards the patient; therefore, self-awareness is paramount. The position and movement of eyes can give insight into the way we are feeling or thinking, whether focusing internally or relating to the environment around us. Eye contact is especially important.

The way in which information is recorded, for example writing notes whilst the assessor is speaking or listening to the patient, could break rapport. The focus and movement of the eyes also give insight into the way people are feeling or thinking, whether they are focusing internally or relating to what is going on around them.

Communication techniques

It may help to identify a specific technique to try to improve communication between health care professionals and patients. An example of one technique is *neurolinguistic programming* (or *NLP*), which can help to identify barriers and assist in overcoming them. Its name comes from the three areas it brings together: *n*eurology, *l*anguage and *p*rogramming.

NLP is a tool that is based on the notion of *well-formed outcomes*, which focuses on positive outcomes and uses the following six-point plan:

1. **Goal:** What do you want?
2. **Evidence:** When will you know you have achieved this?
3. **Specifics:** When, where and how?
4. **Resources:** What resources do you have? What resources will you need?
5. **Ecological:** What are the advantages of making this change? What are the disadvantages of making this change?
6. **Worthwhile:** What is important about you achieving this? What is the benefit of this outcome?

In order for patients to gain control over the process of change and make the journey successful they need to be supported to consider the above. Change is a journey from an unsatisfactory present state to a desired state, an outcome. Various resources are used to make the journey. If used correctly, the continence care pathway is a logical tool for effectively finding a positive outcome for both the health care professional and the patient; therefore, for both, changes will have occurred.

Health care professionals wishing to explore NLP further should refer to *NLP and Coaching for Healthcare Professionals* by Henwood and Lister (2007), published by Wiley-Blackwell.

Using the continence care pathway: examples of NLP

The first part of the pathway identifies the issue and leads the health care professional to the appropriate pathway: stress, urge or overflow. This is where well-formed outcomes can lead to the best outcome for both the health care professional and the patient. For example, after an initial assessment, it is identified that the patient has genuine stress incontinence and starts on the care pathway. Using the six-point plan can clarify the journey for the patient and professional.

1. The goal, positively stated, is that the patient wants to be able to exercise without leakage.
2. The evidence will be that this is achieved and the patient no longer leaks on exertion.
3. Specifics need to be addressed, including how will you do the exercises, when will you do them and how frequently?
4. What resources will be required? Evidence-based and patient-friendly information to support the plan, support in the form of follow-up, or referral to a women's health physiotherapist. Time and motivation.
5. Ecological: advantages could be life-changing.
6. Worthwhile. How important is this outcome to you?

Case histories using NLP techniques

Amanda, aged 50 years, has increasing stress leakage on exertion.

1. The goal was that Amanda wanted to be dry and be able to dance and run without leaking.
2. The evidence will be when she has achieved this.
3. She had identified that she would need to make the exercises a priority, which made her very upset, as she realised that she had the resources to make this change herself. She committed to doing pelvic floor exercises as per her individual plan, twice a day, morning and evening.
4. She was able to use her pelvic floor and wanted to have additional resources for a women's health physiotherapist. She was given written information and follow-up support.
5. The advantages were that she was given a way to achieve her goal and this would improve her confidence; the disadvantages were that she would have to find time and make this a priority in her life.
6. She was clear that this was worthwhile and was very important to her, in order for her to continue the physical activities.

Keith, aged 60 years, with bowel dysfunction after a resection for bowel cancer. He had struggled for a year, spending four hours a night on a commode, watching television, waiting for his bowel to empty completely. He was also wearing pads for faecal leakage.

He had put his social life completely on hold.

1. His goal was to reduce the time spent on the commode, to resume his social life and to be able to go out in the evenings and go on holiday.
2. The evidence would be when he could empty his bowel in half an hour and not leak.
3. He was taught how to use a bowel washout.
4. He was able to use the equipment and had support from the specialist nurses and his partner.
5. The advantages were life-changing: he could empty his bowel in half an hour, had no leakage and no longer needed pads. He was now able to socialise in the evenings, and had regained some dignity in his life for the first time for a year. He was now planning a holiday with his partner.
6. The outcome for him was life-changing. He wrote thanking the specialists: 'Thank you for giving me my life back.'

A positive outcome overcomes barriers to change and can only be achieved when the health care professional fosters a strong rapport with the patient. This will be based on an understanding of how a patient can sense the health care professional's thoughts and feelings – which can influence the outcome of any treatment – and of the way a patient chooses to communicate (body language etc.), which will enable the health care professional to build a better picture of the patient's needs than one based solely upon what the patient says.

A patient who believes that absorbent pads are the only answer will struggle to be motivated to commence pelvic floor exercises or bladder retraining. If the health care professional can guide the patient to consider well-formed outcomes, change in that perception is more likely.

If, after using the pathway, it is decided that pads or appliances are the best outcome, making sure that the correct product is provided is in itself a positive outcome for both the patient and the health care professional.

Language

Language can have an impact on both health and healing, and has the power and impact on our behaviour and response. In health care it is very easy to set up or reinforce negative feelings or set up a negative response. So, for example, saying to the patient 'Tell me about your incontinence' purely reinforces this, and the patient will believe that they are incontinent, with all the connotations that word possesses.

Changing the statement to 'Tell me how your bladder is bothering you' creates a different response, and introduces the concept of incontinence as an issue that can be treated. Changing the way patients are talked to could change the way they talk to themselves (which could be exacerbating their condition) and increase the chance of overcoming the barrier to change. Patients are more likely to talk about *urgency* or *leakage* than *incontinence*. A positive outcome will overcome barriers to change and can only be achieved when the health care professional becomes aware of the communication between themselves and the patient. Using some of the simple tools that exist within NLP will make a difference to the effectiveness of the clinical intervention and achieve a satisfactory outcome for the patient, carer and health care professional. Barriers to change can be overcome, both by the health care professional and by the patient.

Key summary points

- Pathways can be developed as part of service redesign or local adaption.
- Local need, requirements and resources must be taken into account.
- Key stakeholders must be involved.
- Barriers to change can be overcome.
- Good communication improves outcomes and patient satisfaction.
- Patients need to be empowered to control the process of change.

Chapter 4

The generic continence pathway

A generic continence pathway is one that contains standards of care that can be applied to all patients with urinary incontinence, whatever the cause of the problem. It is important that it includes all the local and national standards that are relevant to the group of patients and reflects their needs. For example, for patients who are resident in a nursing home it would be logical to consider the inclusion of statements about nutrition or skin care in vulnerable patients.

The generic care pathway utilises standards, which are a professionally agreed level of care, encapsulating a definition of good practice. The standard is expressed in the form of a statement, against which current practice can be tested to see whether or not the standard has been achieved. A standard statement specifies the most appropriate evidence-based care and the actions that need to be taken if the patient falls outside the standard. The standard must not be idealistic but realistic and achievable.

This chapter covers all the factors of care that the body of evidence suggests are applicable to all individuals whose continence status is at risk, irrespective of age or morbidity. These factors are identified in Figure 4.1. Patient experiences are outlined to help develop the explanation of the standards. The patient experiences have come directly from patients whom the authors have treated in their clinical practice of over 40 years of combined experience. Various administrative data are suggested, but these may be changed to accommodate the needs of the particular client group or management specification.

Figure 4.1 Standards included in a generic pathway

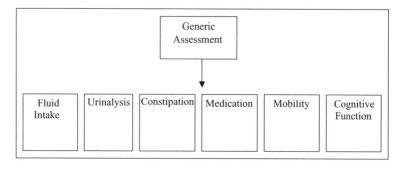

Fluid intake

The first standard statement in the generic pathway relates to fluid intake.

Patient drinks ____ amount of fluid per day.

To help identify the normal parameters a fluid template may specify the amount a person should drink appropriate to their weight or their medical condition.

The layout of the pathway allows for the easy recording of variances. Variances are any deviation from the standard (see Chapter 2). For example, if a patient has been advised by their doctor to reduce their fluid intake due to cardiac failure, then that fact should be recorded in the variance column and signed and dated. Assessing a patient's fluid intake and giving appropriate evidence-based advice is an essential part of a continence assessment. Many patients with urinary incontinence or an overactive bladder will reduce the amount that they drink in the hope that it will improve their problem.

> *I suddenly felt the need to pass urine when I was shopping in the supermarket and wet myself. I have never been so embarrassed in all my life. I do not drink in the mornings now on the days I go shopping. (Mary, aged 75)*

Not drinking enough, especially in older patients, may lead to dehydration, constipation and increases the risk of urinary tract infection (UTI). Concentrated urine is more irritating to the bladder and may increase urinary frequency. It is therefore important that patients be discouraged from restricting fluids in this way; but if they do, they need to make up for the missed fluid when they get home. It is important to maintain hydration as a prevention of constipation (Arnaud, 2003). Excessive fluid intake may also lead to lower-urinary-tract symptoms, such as urinary frequency.

The NICE guidelines *The Management of Urinary Incontinence in Women* (National Institute for Health and Clinical Excellence, 2006) recommends that practitioners consider advising modification of high or low fluid intake for the treatment of women with urinary incontinence or overactive bladder. This advice may also be applied to male patients.

An intake of 1.5 litres of fluid per day should be sufficient for metabolic needs and will maintain sufficiently dilute urine output to avoid the irritation of concentrated urine (Parsons and Cardozo, 2004).

Advice on fluid intake may be influenced by medical conditions, for example a person with chronic renal failure may be advised to reduce their intake, whilst a patient with a UTI will be advised to drink more. If strenuous exercise has been taken or the weather is hot, then the amount needs to be increased.

Some patients do not like drinking water and advice on alternatives like diluted fruit juice, fruit and herbal teas or adding a slice of lemon to the water should be given. Patients should be advised to avoid drinks containing caffeine (this is discussed in detail later). There is anecdotal evidence that fizzy drinks may cause urinary frequency and urgency. It may also be possible to increase the intake by giving more fruit, yoghurt, cereal or soup.

Establishing what patients like to drink and when will encourage increased consumption. Whether people take sugar or like their tea or coffee milky or strong will make all the difference to their actually drinking it. If the patient is unable to provide the information, then relatives or carers may be able to.

No one asked me what I liked to drink with my breakfast when I went into the nursing home, so on the first morning I did not get my usual glass of orange juice. I got really constipated. (Maud, aged 90)

Special drinking cups or something as simple as a drinking straw may mean that the patient can drink independently. If they cannot, then it is vital that all the staff are made aware that the patient will need help.

If a patient is not drinking enough, it is worth exploring why.

Lily, aged 90, was always a tea drinker. When she was admitted to a nursing home, she was leaving her tea. This was because she liked it very hot and the tea that was served was cold. It was decided that she should be given her own pot of tea. After that, she immediately started drinking tea again.

It is recommended that for patients who are in receipt of residential or nursing care or packages of care in their own home a statement be inserted establishing their preferences regarding fluid intake, if this is not documented elsewhere.

It may be helpful to include a statement about the type of fluid drunk as caffeinated or alcoholic drinks may exacerbate symptoms. Alternatively, this may be included in a general information sheet.

Cranberry juice

Patients with continence problems are sometimes told to drink cranberry juice for its therapeutic properties. In fact, it is recommended only for UTI. Cranberries have been used to treat UTI by American Indians for centuries, whilst in recent years cranberry juice has been used in this country to reduce the number of UTIs. Meta-analysis of four trials showed that cranberry products reduced the risk of UTI overall (Jepson and Craig, 2008). It has been shown to decrease the number of infections in women over a 12-month period but will not be effective for all patients. As resistance to antibiotics in patients has increased, the use of cranberry juice, tablets or capsules has grown. They are not a replacement for antibiotics but should be used as appropriate.

Cranberry juice is available widely and is usually sweetened because it has a tart taste. A reduced-sugar drink is also available. It is most beneficial to purchase the cranberry juice with the highest juice content. It can be purchased mixed with other juices, such as raspberry. Cranberry may be bought as both tablets and capsules from health food shops. If patients do not like the taste of the juice, they may find tablets or capsules more palatable. The recommended amount of juice is 300 ml daily (Avorn et al., 1994). Compounds found in cranberry fruit prevent antibiotic-resistant and susceptible uropathogenic bacteria from attaching to uroepithelial cells, preventing them from multiplying and causing infection. The antibacterial adhesion effect persists in human urine for up to 10 hours following ingestion of cranberry juice (Howell *et al.*, 1998). As UTIs develop rapidly, it needs to be taken on a regular daily basis; just missing one day may be all that is needed to allow an infection to return.

I had suffered from cystitis for years, and so was advised to drink cranberry juice twice a day. I have not had an infection for at least 12 months. (Jane, aged 34)

The juice is recommended for patients who suffer from cystitis, UTI, stone formation or have mucus in their urine. Cranberry juice is not suitable for all patients (Leaver, 1996). As cranberry juice is acidic, it is not recommended for patients who have gastric ulcers or for those who suffer from gastritis. Diabetics should be made aware that it contains sugar, and should seek medical advice before taking it. Cranberry juice interacts with warfarin and should not be taken by patients on this or any other anti-coagulant therapy.

Caffeine

In patients who are susceptible caffeine intake may cause frequency of urination and an urgent need to void. Many patients suffering from these symptoms will experience improvement in their symptoms if they eliminate caffeine from their diet. If a patient does have a large intake, the NICE guideline recommends a trial of caffeine reduction, as this may reduce urinary frequency and urgency (National Institute for Health and Clinical Excellence, 2006).

Caffeine is a drug which is found in tea, coffee, cocoa, chocolate and cola. It is also used in a range of painkillers and cold remedies. Caffeine is a stimulant which acts directly on the heart and central nervous system. It can increase alertness but also causes insomnia. People who have a regular intake of caffeine may become addicted. However, even a relatively low caffeine intake will affect the bladder of a susceptible person.

Users of caffeinated drinks and food types will often feel the effects of caffeine withdrawal. Symptoms can be in the form of headache, anxiety, difficulty in concentrating, drowsiness and muscular stiffness. The most common symptom is headache, which is reported by 50% of people who withdraw from caffeine use (Anon, 2004).

Many people report a very good success ratio by cutting down caffeine at the rate of 50–100 mg per day. This is known as *caffeine fading*. The best way to proceed is to write down the caffeine intake for one week, then reduce the caffeine intake as above. Withdrawal symptoms are more marked if caffeine is eliminated from the diet without fading. Regular caffeine consumption reduces sensitivity to caffeine. When intake is reduced, the body becomes oversensitive to adenosine. As a response to this, the blood pressure drops dramatically, leading to a headache. This usually lasts from one to five days and can be alleviated with painkillers, so long as those which include caffeine are avoided. This headache, which is well known amongst strong and heavy coffee drinkers, will also be alleviated by an intake of caffeine. In research (Stavric *et al.*, 1988) abstinence from doses as low as 100 mg per day produced symptoms, but generally the higher the consumption, the more likely you are to have withdrawal symptoms.

Urinary symptoms will regress within a week or so. It will help to keep a diary of symptoms for comparative purposes.

> *I tried to go caffeine-free, but I got a terrible headache, felt awful and even my legs hurt. I used caffeine fading instead and still felt rough but managed to get through it. I don't have to go to the toilet half as much as I used to and I feel better as well. (Anna, aged 41)*

Suggested standard statements which may form part of the generic pathway

Urinalysis

Urinalysis performed: if nitrite or leucocyte are present or symptoms of urinary infection, take midstream specimen of urine and discontinue pathway until treated.

Urinary tract infection (UTI) is the second most common clinical indication for empirical antimicrobial treatment in primary and secondary care and urine samples constitute the largest single category of specimens examined in most microbiology laboratories (Scottish Intercollegiate Guidelines Network, 2004). Urinalysis using a reagent strip needs to be carried out on all patients as part of their initial continence assessment (Figure 4.2). This will not only ensure that any patient with a UTI is identified and appropriate treatment is given but will also screen for other diseases such as diabetes and help in the managing and planning of care. An older person may suddenly appear confused and/or incontinent of urine without apparent reason or having any of the typical symptoms of a UTI, but it is always worth testing their urine for exclusion (Richards, 2008).

The best urine specimen is one voided first thing in the morning. This is because it is at its most concentrated and has been in the bladder for four hours, which makes it optimal for testing because it takes this time for nitrate to convert to nitrite. Random samples may be used, but sensitivity will be lower. It should be voided into a clean, dry receptacle or collected in a sterile container. It then needs to be tested within four hours of collection. It may be stored in a refrigerator if not tested within one hour, but needs to return to room temperature for testing.

Specimens may also be collected from babies or adults who are incontinent using a urine collection pack. The pack contains:

■ two small pads
■ 5 ml syringe
■ one sterile specimen container.

A pad is placed over the area where the patient passes urine and is frequently checked to see whether it is wet. A wet pad is removed and laid on a flat surface, wet side up. The syringe tip is placed at an angle of 45 degrees and urine extracted from the pad and placed in the sterile container.

Normal urine should appear clear and pale yellow in colour, whilst concentrated urine will be a deeper yellow. Infected urine will be cloudy and may contain blood. Uninfected urine is odourless, whilst infected urine will have an offensive smell. Patients with a UTI may complain of dysuria, urinary frequency and urgency as well as backache and of generally feeling unwell.

There are many different types of reagent strips available. NICE recommends that testing should include tests for blood, glucose, protein, leucocytes and nitrite (National Institute for Health and Clinical Excellence, 2006). It is imperative that the reagent strip

Figure 4.2   An example of a generic pathway

Urinary Continence Care Pathway Assessment

Full name:		Date of birth:
Address:		Postcode:
		Tel:
GP:	Practice:	NHS number:
Assessor:	Designation:	Tel:

What has been the effect of your bladder problem on your life?

How much does it bother you? (Tick your choice or give ICIQ score.)

....

A lot ☐   *moderately* ☐   *a little* ☐   *not at all* ☐

Standard statement	Variance from standard statement and reason/comments
Patient drinks _____ amount of fluid per day	
If patient drinks caffeinated or alcoholic drinks, advice/general information sheet provided	
If patient drinks volumes outside of recommended template, advise them to drink appropriate amount unless they have been advised otherwise for medical reasons	
Urinalysis performed:	
Glucose		
Ketone	
S. gravity	
Blood	
PH	
Protein	
Nitrite	
Leucocytes	
If leucocytes/nitrite or symptoms of urinary infection present, take MSU and discontinue this assessment until treated	
Patient reports no symptoms of constipation or signs and symptoms chart completed using Stool Chart. Consider use of Bowel Care Pathway.	

Standard statement	Variance from standard statement and reason/comments
Patient is not taking medication on list provided or consider for review	
Patient has no mobility dexterity or environmental problems, or record any action taken	
Patient has no signs of cognitive dysfunction or give 'Continence in the Confused elderly' sheet to patient/carer	
Symptom Profile completed by patient	
Patient commenced on appropriate colour-coded care pathway as indicated from Symptom Profile	

This patient is unable to commence on a CP because:

TO BE COMPLETED BY ALL STAFF USING THE PATHWAY
Sign to confirm that you have met all standards or recorded variances

Full name	Designation	Initials	Sign	Date

is read correctly. Nurses have many demands on their time but need to be aware that it will take two minutes to get an accurate reading. Failure to allow enough time may result in a false reading of negative for nitrite and leucocytes, the indicators for urinary tract infection.

Leucocytes

Infections of the urinary tract usually produce pus cells. These release an esterase that reacts with the reagent pad. The presence of leucocytes in the urine is an indication of bladder or renal infection. A positive result indicates the need for urine to be sent for microscopy, culture and sensitivity.

Nitrite

Nitrite is not a normal constituent of urine, so when it is found there is always an infection present. Most of the organisms which infect the urinary tract contain an enzyme system that catalyses the conversion of nitrate. Urine should be sent for culture and microscopy. False negatives include lack of incubation in the bladder. The ideal specimen should have been in the bladder for at least four hours. This provides time for the nitrate–nitrite conversion. Negative results should always be viewed in the light of other test results.

Blood

Presence of blood in the urine suggests serious renal or urological disease and/or urine infection. Follow-up will depend on the results from other tests and the clinical picture.

Protein

Transient positive tests are seldom important. Persistent positive test results indicate renal disease, UTI, hypertension, pre-eclampsia or congestive cardiac failure. The nitrite, blood and leucocyte results should always be noted in this case.

> I went to see my GP because I had a urine infection. They tested my urine and said it was all right. I had to go back again because I did have an infection. They said it was because I had drunk a lot to try to get rid of the infection. (Margaret, aged 40)

A false negative can occur if patients drink a large amount, as it dilutes the specimen.

Urinalysis is an essential part of a continence assessment. It is a quick and easy means of screening for infection. It is cost-effective and reduces the need for unnecessary laboratory testing whilst informing the process of care planning.

Constipation

Patient reports no symptoms of constipation, or Signs and Symptoms Chart completed using Stool Chart.

Constipation is a very common problem, especially in older patients. Constipation may predispose patients to urinary incontinence and, in women, to urogenital prolapse (National Institute for Health and Clinical Excellence, 2006).

The causes and treatment of constipation are dealt with both in this chapter and in Chapter 6. In this chapter the reader will find detailed data on environmental factors, including mobility, and some information on diet and medication, which is further discussed in Chapter 6, which deals with designing a bowel care pathway. Faecal incontinence is also dealt with separately. However, the issue of constipation will also be addressed in this section as it is a significant cause of urinary incontinence and will certainly exacerbate the symptoms.

The cause of constipation is the large bolus of faeces sitting just behind and pressing directly on the bladder wall. It is very important that patients understand the anatomy and physiology behind the mechanics of constipation, as much of the advice given to alleviate the symptoms and prevent reoccurrence is not always welcome. Chapter 6 also contains additional information, including the physiology of the bowel, other causes of constipation and treatments.

However, it is important to establish at this point just what is meant by *constipation*. Many eminent physicians have tried to define this. There are many people, particularly older people, who will claim that they are constipated if they miss a single day, and some people are concerned if they do not have their bowels open at the same time every day. The concerns are not always time- or regularity-focused. If a patient has to strain or if the consistency of the stool has changed, they may consider themselves constipated.

The recommended standard diagnostic criterion for functional incontinence is two or more episodes for at least three months of:

- straining at defecation at least a quarter of the time
- lumpy and hard stools at least a quarter of the time
- a sensation of incomplete evacuation at least a quarter of the time
- two or fewer bowel motions in a week.

(Thompson *et al.*, 1999, cited in Norton and Chelvanayagam, 2004)

It is imperative to establish with each individual what they would describe as being constipated and what, in their opinion, is normal. Whatever the setting for patients this is a vital starting point.

Depending on the cohort of patients in this setting, standard statements could establish when they last had their bowels opened, a Stool Chart rating and whether they consider themselves constipated and why.

Again, the recommendation is that people are adequately hydrated (Arnaud, 2003), and unless there is clear understanding about the role of the large bowel in the reabsorbing of water then patients are unlikely to comply. The setting in which the pathway is to be used is critical. For those using pathways with a group of fast-throughput secondary care sector patients it may simply be that, as part of the pathway, maintaining an adequate fluid intake may be as much as can be achieved. However, in a longer-stay environment it will be very important to establish individual likes and dislikes, as previously stated. A care pathway designed around the prevention and treatment of constipation could be invaluable in this type of setting.

It is well established that diet has a huge impact on constipation. A diet high in both soluble and non-soluble fibre will go a long way to preventing a recurrence of bouts of constipation. However, it is not easy to get people to change their diets. Many who are chronically constipated are older people, who often do not wish to vary their diet.

> I'm 91 and live alone and my food is the one thing left for me to enjoy. I'm not going to eat brown bread and brown rice at my time of life. My appetite isn't that good and I'm going to eat what I like. (Mary Ann, aged 91)

Many older people have to rely upon others to do their shopping or cannot afford to spend too much money on food they may not like. They may also see recommendations about certain food groups as the latest fashion, with research presenting various foods as healthy or unhealthy on a weekly basis.

> My dad ate toast and dripping and meat fat all his life and he was 90 when he died. He never had any problems. (Phoebe, aged 84)

It will be necessary therefore to spend some time with this cohort of patients, not trying to change their routine or lifestyles but identifying what foods which are higher in fibre they do like to eat and encouraging those. It must be noted that if non-soluble fibre foods are increased then the fluid intake must be adequate to compensate for this; otherwise, the constipation may become worse.

Many patients in long-term care suffer from constipation, and it is harder to individualise their care. However, it could be useful to discuss with the patient first which fruits, biscuits or cakes they are most likely to eat and to tailor these to their needs (for example fruit cake rather than sponge). When recommending a change in diet, it is important to ensure that false teeth or plates are comfortable, as many of the recommended foods can cause pain if caught under a plate or are simply not easy to eat with dentures in situ.

I used to love raspberries, but I can't eat them now. The pips get under my plate. I wouldn't dare risk an apple. My late husband used to peel one for me and quarter it. I could eat it then, but I haven't had one since he died. (Sylvia, aged 87)

The use of laxatives for treatment purposes is discussed fully in Chapter 6. However, many people have self-medicated throughout their lives and, as mentioned previously, it is often the understanding of the definition of constipation that drives this. Some older patients feel that they need regular laxatives to clear themselves out.

We always had syrup of figs on a Friday night. We had to stand in line, and Mum used the same teaspoon for all of us. (Emma, aged 87)

It is important to obtain a history of self-medication before decisions can be made, and a standard statement relating to this should be an integral part of a constipation pathway.

The environment surrounding the toilet is very important. In their own home most people have heating, good lighting, soft and often moist toilet paper, a good book or newspaper and adequate privacy. This must be replicated as far as possible in a care setting. People especially need privacy to have their bowels opened satisfactorily, and this requires both visual privacy – a locked door, preferably not of the cubicle variety – and aural privacy, with others around not being able to hear. This can be achieved at least in part where it is not possible to provide by turning on a radio or television to mask sounds. Establish what the routine at home was, using a standard statement, and attempt to replicate as far as is possible.

My mum never let me sit on a public toilet seat so I always squat over it. I couldn't bring myself to sit on it so when I was in hospital I just didn't go for five days. (Sonya, aged 49)

I was OK until I had my first baby, then it hurt so much that I didn't go for ages and I've never been quite right since. (Jackie, aged 42)

When designing the pathway, it is strongly advised that a basic information sheet(s) be provided that targets the particular group of patients with the information most likely to help them.

Medication

Patient is not taking medication on list provided, or consider referral to GP for review.

This section concentrates on the side effects of medication and the impact on continence. Many different types of medication may affect continence status in different ways and it is important to consider the effects of pharmacy. Again, when localising pathways, medications which are common to individual patient groups such as mental health or neurological dysfunction may be specifically included. It may be that medications can be manipulated or alternatives tried, but it may simply be that having identified the cause of a symptom it can be managed. Medication side effects are shown in Appendix 2, Information sheet 3.

Environmental factors

Patient has no mobility dexterity or environmental problems, or record any action taken.

The NHS Plan (Department of Health, 2000a) reinforced the importance of getting the basics right and of improving patient experience. The *Essence of Care* (Department of Health, 2001) provided a tool to help practitioners take a patient-focused and structured approach to sharing and comparing practice. This resulted in benchmarks covering a number of areas of care.

The benchmarks, Continence and Bladder and Bowel Care, Privacy and Dignity are inter-related and important (Department of Health 2001). Best practice demands that the environment is adapted to meet the individual needs of patients and that consultation with specialist continence professionals has taken place in assessing the environment. Environmental problems that affect continence may be related to:

■ mobility
■ manual dexterity
■ transferring
■ personal care.

There are thousands of products available and solutions to these problems. The professionals who can help and give advice are occupational therapists and physiotherapists, who may be based in a hospital, rehabilitation unit or in the community. There are also specialist centres that provide free advice on independent living equipment, such as Assist UK, which is a national network of centres for advice on independent living equipment. The centres provide free advice and information, and people can try out a wide range of products and find solutions to problems.

One occupational therapist at a centre describes that, owing to embarrassment, people rarely make an appointment for a continence problem, but will mention it if asked during an assessment if they have any other problems. Referral is open so that people can refer themselves or come with a relative or a professional, such as a community occupational therapist.

Mary, 55 years old, was weight bearing but unable to get herself off the toilet. An electronic toilet lift solved the problem. Phyllis, a 75-year-old lady with severe arthritis, was given advice about a lightweight raised toilet seat that she could take on holiday with her. David, who was 45 years old and suffered from multiple sclerosis, used a male urinal at night but frequently spilled the contents when trying to remove it. A non-spill adaptor fitted into the urinal was all that was needed.

These centres do not sell equipment but can give people advice on where best to obtain it and ensure that it is the best solution for the problem. They are also able to give advice on what is supplied free or if and where grants may be obtained.

Gwen an 85-year-old lady who had the misfortune to trip over her bedspread in her bedroom at home and fractured her femur. She was admitted to her district general hospital and underwent a total hip replacement. After a few days she was well enough to be transferred to her local cottage hospital.

The aim was for Gwen to be able to get out of bed, dress herself and walk to the toilet unaided. To be able to do this she would needed to:

1. get out of bed
2. transfer to her chair
3. dress herself
4. walk to the toilet
5. sit on the toilet
6. wipe her bottom
7. get up from the toilet
8. adjust her clothing
9. wash her hands
10. walk back to her chair.

The ward physiotherapist and occupational therapist were the professionals who helped Gwen to achieve this. Both were aware of the range of equipment available and were able to give advice and, in some cases, provide Gwen with what was needed.

She was able to get herself to the side of the bed with the help of a walking frame, which had been adjusted to the correct height by the physiotherapist. The physiotherapist supervised her transfer to the chair, again at the right height for Gwen. There are many different hoists, rails, boards, risers and poles that could have been used if needed and the therapists would assess her needs and recommend the best solution. When it came to dressing, the occupational therapist gave Gwen a device to help her put on her stockings and a long-handled shoehorn to provide the reach she needed to put on her slippers. Had it been necessary, Gwen could have been given a catalogue of clothing designed for people with disabilities. For example, garments have elasticised waists, or zips and buttons replaced by Velcro. In some areas there are clothing services that will give advice or alter or adapt clothing for a small charge.

Gwen was able under the supervision of the physiotherapist to walk to the toilet. An alternative might have been for Gwen to use a commode. There is a vast range of commodes available with or without wheels. Special features, such as folding arms, height adjustment and comfort seats, can be obtained. Commodes can be made of metal, plastic or wood and even look like an ordinary chair. Extra-wide commodes are also available. An occupational therapist would be able to assess and advise on the most suitable one for each patient.

The toilet was equipped with an adjustable toilet surround, a raised toilet seat and grab rails. Gwen, with the help of these, was able to sit on the toilet and pass urine, having adjusted her clothing.

She was able to wipe her bottom but had she not been able to there are a number of bottom wipers that she could have used. Several may need to be tried because, for example, someone with rheumatoid arthritis may find one easier to use than another. An automatic toilet that provides flushing warm water and warm-air drying could provide another solution. Getting off the toilet may be difficult for some patients and a toilet lift designed to lower or raise a patient on or off the toilet may be needed.

When equipment is supplied, it is important to consider the whole problem. There is no point in supplying a commode if there is no one available to empty it. This solves one problem whilst creating another.

Gwen was able to return to her home. Being mobile and able to toilet herself were important factors in Gwen being able to return home; otherwise, the alternative might have been long-term care.

Cognitive dysfunction

Patient has no signs of cognitive dysfunction, or give information sheet on cognitive sheet to patient/carer.

The way we stay continent is a very complex function that allows us to voluntarily postpone passing urine or having our bowels opened until we are at the appropriate place. This skill is something that can be affected by a dementing illness.

Alzheimer's disease is an illness disabling the cognitive, functional and behavioural domains that affect the ability to maintain continence. The interdependency of these domains can magnify the efforts required to maintain continence.

It may happen just occasionally or, as the illness progresses, more frequently. It is very important to try to help the patient keep their continence skills for as long as possible, as this may be the precipitating factor that precedes long-term care.

Lack of recall may also mean they gradually lose the memory of what to do in a toilet or even where the toilet is. Repetition is extremely important in maintaining continence skills for those people whose cognitive function is diminishing.

It may also be that the person finds it difficult to verbally pass on the information of the need to use a toilet. If this is the case, it is important to become aware of verbal or behavioural cues, such as fidgeting, wandering or pulling at clothing. Obviously, this entails considerable observation of the person. It can help to keep a behavioural record so that the signs that predispose to a bladder or bowel movement can be ascertained. Clear signage can also be helpful as a reminder. It must be noted that the continence status of a person with cognitive dysfunction rests on a knife edge and can be very easily tipped into incontinence.

I could manage until he went into respite. We had a routine. When he came back, he was wearing a pad and he's worn one ever since. Trouble is, now he's started to take them off. (Mrs H, looking after her elderly husband)

Whilst it is clear that carers need breaks from care, it is imperative to try to maintain whatever routine they have established. If a home diary can be kept prior to any admission, discussed with a primary carer and forms the core of the care plan, then continence is much more likely to be maintained. Moreover, advice should be given also to any informal carer.

I went to France for four days for a break and my daughter came to look after him. She knew what to do: she's a nurse. When I came back, he'd been picking at his bottom and his nails were full of poo. She didn't know I gave him baby wipes every time he went to the loo. I suppose he felt itchy and now he's sore. He's still doing it. (Mrs C regarding her husband, aged 85)

Communication between formal and informal carers is essential. Sequencing can be very helpful, where small, everyday tasks are broken down into individual pieces, much as in the mapping process described in Chapter 3.

Hutchinson *et al.* (1996) describe 21 steps needed for successful self-toileting (Box 4.1).

Box 4.1   Steps for successful self-toileting

- Recognising the urge to go
- Going to bathroom by self or requesting assistance or going when asked
- Closing the door
- Pulling pants down/unzipping trousers
- Sitting on toilet or pulling penis out
- Void or have bowel movement
- Get toilet paper
- Wiping
- Putting paper in toilet
- Standing up, putting penis in pants
- Flushing
- Pulling up pants/zipping pants
- Turn on tap
- Washing hands
- Using soap
- Turning off tap
- Getting towel
- Drying hands
- Putting towel in bin/replacing towel
- Leaving bathroom
- Closing door

They go on to describe instances of distraction that will interfere with the completion of the whole task. If it is possible to observe the individual, it may be that the steps that are causing the most problems can be identified and solved. It can be seen very clearly that this step process will change considerably depending on the environment, and therefore why repetition and replication are so pivotal in maintaining continence. The person must also feel secure in the environment. They may refuse to use the toilet because the environment is not what they are used to or because they feel unsafe. This also demonstrates the importance of communication between family and formal and informal carers.

Whilst any generic care pathway must include cognitive function, the width and breadth of information can only be decided locally by a pathway implementation group, which designs pathways for its particular patient cohort. Those who are working directly with people with cognitive dysfunction may prefer to write a separate pathway having used a mini mental score to ascertain levels of dysfunction. This could be based on the steps required for successful toileting.

For those providing care in a more general environment, an information sheet may be provided if necessary, including local information and sources of help and support, or a referral if certain criteria are met. The mapping process will help this considerably.

Key summary points

- Fluid intake is a critical component of continence care.
- Urinalysis must always be performed.
- Constipation must be excluded.
- Medication should be reviewed.
- Environmental issues can resolve continence problems.
- Cognitive dysfunction must be considered in its own right.

Chapter 5

Symptom-related specific pathways

The generic pathway is suitable for all patients, irrespective of age, clinical condition and cognitive function. However, in order to meet individual clinical need, developing pathways that are condition-specific can be very helpful. There are many ways in which these can be approached. They can be symptom-related, as for stress urge and overflow incontinence, or diagnostically related, as for multiple sclerosis. In this chapter it is intended to give an overview of how care pathways can be put together and examples of the symptom profile that may be used to identify which type of incontinence a person is suffering from. This will be followed by the specific pathways for each type and actions to take. For each statement given the evidence is provided to make it easier for the potential pathway designer to use.

Diagnostic pathways have the advantage of the patient already being diagnosed, and therefore the disease process and the related continence problems will have some predictability. It is essential, for example, to undertake assessment of residual urine and voiding difficulties in a patient with neurological dysfunction. A history may provide evidence of repeated urine infection. For a patient who is compliant and able, this points to intermittent self-catheterisation, and a pathway can be designed to accommodate this. However, great care should be taken in the pathway to ensure correct diagnosis, as other conditions can mimic these symptoms but are treated in a different manner. Diagnostic pathways will be mainly used by nurses caring for specific groups of patients, and here we intend to concentrate on symptom-related pathways.

Quality of life

It is important at this juncture to recognise the importance of measuring the quality of life of those patients who suffer from incontinence. In 1998 the Scientific Committee of the International Continence Society recognised the need to develop a universally applicable questionnaire for wide application across international populations in clinical practice and research to assess urinary incontinence, facilitating the comparison of findings from different settings and studies, in a manner similar to the International Prostate Symptom Score. The first module developed was the International Consultation on Incontinence Modular Questionnaire (ICIQ) short-form questionnaire for urinary incontinence. ICIQ modules have been developed or adapted for urinary tract symptoms, and modules to assess patient satisfaction are of particular use for assessing treatment effectiveness (Avery *et al.*, 2004). This can be obtained by using the ICIQ LUTS profile, which has a possible bothersome rating of 120. The aim is to reduce the bothersome rating for the patient even if the symptoms do not improve, enabling them to manage their symptoms more effectively and improve their quality of life. For those professionals dealing with incontinence symptoms it is essential to identify whether the quality of life has improved. Many patients will not necessarily get an overall improvement in their symptoms or may have intractable incontinence. However, helping them to manage this will improve their quality of life considerably, and it is essential to measure the impact that contact with a health professional has made. The ICIQ questionnaires are strongly recommended. For more information visit http://www.ICIQ.net.

Symptom profile, assessment and standard statements

Care pathways for this purpose are assuming no particular skills in continence care, and therefore it is necessary that the data collected assist the health care professional in making the jump from assessment to diagnosis. A self-administered symptom profile can be used to assess the type of incontinence and can be colour-coded to the appropriate pathway. This profile contains a set of questions for each symptom, depending on the number of symptoms identified, and these could include:

- stress
- urge/urgency
- voiding dysfunction/overflow
- nocturia
- cystitis
- nocturnal enuresis
- diurnal enuresis
- cognitive dysfunction
- catheterisation
- intermittent self-catheterisation.

It is intended here to concentrate on the stress, urge and overflow pathways, as these were the original pathways identified by the authors as the most frequently occurring symptoms. Therefore, three sets of questions have been identified. Using the available evidence to support each component, the authors used the symptom profile shown in Figure 5.1.

This profile is completed by the patient. This will identify the predominant symptom, leading to the appropriate coloured pathway.

The symptom profile, as well as each of the three pathways and the continence assessment, were peer-reviewed using a method of content validation described by Lynn (1986). This validation process is carried out as means of checking what was produced, by using twelve independent experts, in this instance, practising professionals in continence care. This determines the content representativeness and relevance of the items of an instrument by the application of a judgement process.

The experts were asked to rank the relevance of statements/questions within the paperwork to continence care using a score from 1 to 4, where 1 was deemed not relevant and 4 was very relevant and succinct. The number of experts that had to respond positively to an item/whole pathway for it to be validated was calculated using the Content Validity Index (Lynn, 1986). The respondents also produced written comments that the Continence Development Group found extremely useful in reviewing the paperwork. The results of this peer review are detailed in the Chapter 7.

Figure 5.1 Symptom profile

I leak when I laugh, cough, sneeze, run or jump.	☐
I only ever leak a little urine.	☐
At night I only use the toilet once or not at all.	☐
I always know when I have leaked.	☐
I leak without feeling the need to empty my bladder.	☐
Only my pants get wet when I leak (not outer clothing) or I sometimes wear a panty liner.	☐
I feel a sudden strong urge to pass urine and have to go quickly.	☐
I feel a strong uncontrolled need to pass urine prior to leaking.	☐
I leak moderate or large amounts of urine before I reach the toilet.	☐
I feel that I pass urine frequently.	☐
I get up at night to pass urine at least twice.	☐
I think I had bladder problems as a child.	☐
I find it hard to start to pass urine.	☐
I have to push or strain to pass urine.	☐
My urine flow stops and starts several times.	☐
My urine stream is weaker and slower than it used to be.	☐
I feel that it takes me a long time to empty my bladder.	☐
I feel as if my bladder is not completely empty after I have been to the toilet.	☐
I leak a few drops of urine on to my underwear just after I have passed urine.	☐

Standard statements relating to stress incontinence

Patients entering onto this pathway will have already been screened by the generic pathway and have symptoms of stress urinary incontinence. Therefore, the pathway commences with a bothersome rating.

Box 5.1 Definition of stress incontinence

> *Stress incontinence is the commonest symptom with which women present and is indicated by the involuntary loss of urine during physical exertion. (Laycock and Haslam, 2002)*
>
> *Clinical history alone can correctly diagnose a large proportion of women with USI. (Martin et al., 2006)*

Examples of statements that may be included in a symptom profile of stress incontinence (Box 5.1) are:

I leak when I laugh, cough, sneeze, run or jump.

Involuntary loss of urine during physical exercise is the commonest symptom that women present with. It is usually provoked by coughing, sneezing, running or jumping (Laycock and Haslam, 2002). It can also rarely affect men as a result of prostatectomy or chronic urinary retention (Getliffe and Dolman, 2003). It is also possible for a movement or a cough to result in leakage because of detrusor instability. It is important to distinguish stress incontinence from detrusor instability, as the treatment differs for both types.

I only ever leak a little urine.

The urine lost in stress incontinence is usually in small amounts. It is associated with a smaller volume loss than urge incontinence (Cardozo *et al.*, 2006).

At night I only use the toilet once or not at all.

Nocturia, the complaint of having to wake at night one or more times to void, is not associated with stress incontinence (National Institute for Health and Clinical Excellence, 2006).

I always know when I have leaked.

Patients with stress incontinence know when they have leaked, as the leakage occurs in relation to the physical activity, and are aware at the point of leakage (Roe, 1992).

I leak without feeling the need to empty my bladder.

As stress incontinence is the involuntary loss of urine on exertion, it is not associated with the urge to void (Cardozo *et al.*, 2006).

Only my pants get wet when I leak (not outer clothing) or I sometimes wear a panty liner.

The small leak caused by stress incontinence is absorbed by a panty liner or only wets the patient's pants. Larger leaks are associated with urge incontinence. However, a patient can get quite wet if the trigger for leakage is repeated, such as horse riding or continuous coughing.

Standard statements relating to urge incontinence

Examples of statements that may be included in a symptom profile of urge incontinence (Box 5.2) are:

I feel a sudden strong urge to pass urine and have to go quickly.

Patients with urge incontinence usually complain of urgency with little or no warning of the need to void and may be incontinent before reaching the toilet (Getliffe and Dolman, 2003).

I feel a strong uncontrolled need to pass urine prior to leaking.

Often urine is lost involuntarily before the patient is able to get to the bathroom (Marcell *et al.*, 2003). The symptom of urge

Box 5.2   Definition of urge incontinence

Urge urinary incontinence is the complaint of involuntary leakage accompanied by, or immediately preceded by, a strong desire to void. (Parsons and Cardozo, 2004)

Urge incontinence can to triggered by running water, coughing or simply entering the bathroom. (Laycock and Haslam, 2002)

incontinence is the complaint of involuntary leakage accompanied or preceded by urgency (Abrams *et al.*, 2002).

I leak moderate or large amounts of urine before I reach the toilet.

Loss of the entire contents of the bladder can occur, but the leak will be significantly larger than that felt with stress or overflow incontinence (Marcell *et al.*, 2003). The loss may be partial or complete and will often depend on how fast the sufferer can move and how fast they can get to the nearest toilet (Norton, 1996).

I feel that I pass urine frequently.

Urgency describes an intense desire to void immediately. It often accompanies frequency (Getliffe and Dolman, 2003).

I get up to pass urine at least twice.

Nocturia is usually associated with urge incontinence (Srikrishna *et al.*, 2007).

I think I had bladder problems as a child.

Studies have shown that the cause of these problems may be due to urge incontinence (Getliffe and Dolman, 2003). This may result in significantly later nocturnal enuresis and/or diurnal enuresis in childhood.

Standard statements relating to overflow incontinence

Examples of statements that may be included in a symptom profile of overflow incontinence (Box 5.3) are:

I find it hard to start to pass urine.

Overflow incontinence is associated with hesitancy. Hesitancy is having to wait for the flow to start (Norton, 1996).

Box 5.3 Definition of overflow incontinence

Overflow incontinence secondary to chronic retention of urine is characterised by voiding difficulties, impaired bladder sensation, recurrent urinary tract infections, and the frequent leakage of small amounts of urine. (Laycock and Haslam, 2002)

I have to push or strain to pass urine.

Straining, having to use abdominal effort or manual expression (applying pressure above the pubic bone), may be necessary to empty the bladder (Norton, 1996).

My urine stream is weaker and slower than it used to be.

Outflow obstruction is associated with hesitancy, poor urinary stream and post-micturition dribble (Roe, 1992). Overflow incontinence is characterised by voiding difficulties and impaired bladder sensation (Laycock and Haslam, 2002).

I feel that it takes me a long time to empty my bladder.

Reduced urine flow can be caused by reduced voided urine, bladder outlet obstruction or reduced bladder contractibility (Bourcier et al., 2004).

I feel as if my bladder is not completely empty after I have been to the toilet.

Some people feel that they never completely empty the bladder but are unable to pass the rest, however much they try (Norton, 1996).

I leak a few drops of urine onto my underwear just after I have passed urine.

In some men incontinence takes the form of post-micturition dribbling. A small amount of urine is passed, usually without much sensation, up to several minutes after micturition is complete (Norton, 1996).

Having identified the type – or in the case of mixed urinary incontinence the types – of incontinence a patient is suffering from, it is possible to select the pathway most suitable for the patient. In the case of urinary incontinence the authors identified three: stress, urge and overflow. As each pathway stands alone and users may wish to use only one, where data are the same for standard statements they have been repeated in each pathway.

Treatment options

The severity of the symptoms is not a sufficient indicator on its own of treatment preference and decisions. Treatment should focus more on patients' goals in relation to their lifestyle targets and ambitions (Cardozo *et al.*, 2006). The following paragraphs describe the various treatment options.

■ Pelvic floor exercises are often the first approach combined with advice about diet, fluid, weight loss and reducing smoking. Hay-Smith and Dumoulin (2006) found that pelvic floor exercises helped all women who suffered from incontinence, and those who had stress incontinence and exercised for at least three month benefited the most. Many studies have demonstrated the benefits of pelvic floor exercises but for them to be effective the patient must be able to contract the appropriate muscles and comply with a pelvic floor exercise regimen (Laycock and Haslam, 2002).

■ The pelvic floor educator is a vaginal indicator of pelvic floor contraction, which patients can take home and practise with. It appears to be a useful adjunct to teaching pelvic floor exercises, although no research currently supports its use.

■ Electrical stimulation delivering a current intensity sufficient to depolarise sensory and motor nerves can be used to strengthen striated muscles in the treatment of stress incontinence and normalise micturition reflexes in the treatment of detrusor overactivity and retention (Laycock and Haslam, 2002). A specialist may provide treatment, or a small portable unit may be given to the patient to use at home.

■ Biofeedback may be used to teach the patient how to isolate the pelvic floor muscle and helps to motivate, and electromyography (EMG) will indicate the efficiency of the neuromusculature. It measures the electrical activity of the pelvic floor muscle. It is a useful method which allows patients to see on a screen and hear through an audible signal that they are correctly contracting their pelvic floor muscles.

■ Weighted vaginal cones are another conservative treatment. A weighted cone is placed in the vagina and the pelvic floor muscle contracts to try to keep it in place. A number of different weights are available so that the patient can progress to the next weight. There is no research, however, that demonstrates that cones are significantly better than pelvic floor exercises alone.

■ There are various medications available for urgency and urge incontinence. NICE (National Institute for Health and Clinical Excellence, 2006) suggests that the most cost-effective method is a trial with short-acting oxybutynin, although this may have unwanted side effects such as dry mouth, gastrointestinal disturbances and blurred vision. Other anti-muscarinic medications are available and it is suggested that careful monitoring of patients taking these medications will improve both compliance and effectiveness. Identifying those people for whom the side effects outweigh the benefits and either titrating the dose or changing to a different drug can improve their outcome.

Surgical treatment: a variety of operations is available and the operation of choice is based upon many factors, including general health, age, weight, previous operations and other personal circumstances. Some examples are tension-free vaginal tape, colposuspension and slings, and bulking agents such as collagen.

Stress incontinence care pathways

Stress incontinence is characterised by leakage when you laugh, cough or sneeze, run or jump. It is very common in women and can be caused or aggravated by childbirth, being overweight, constipation and by chronic coughing. It is caused by an incompetent bladder neck closure often weakened during childbirth and made worse by atrophic changes after the menopause, when hormone levels fall. Men may also develop stress incontinence after prostatic surgery (DuBeau *et al.*, 1998). Figure 5.2 gives an example of a stress incontinence care pathway.

Bothersome rating

Patients are asked their bothersome rating at each visit to check whether they are subjectively improving (Bayliss *et al.*, 2000a). The authors used a simple Likert scale. However, it is recommended that users consider using the ICIQ questionnaires discussed earlier in this chapter, as a specific score/rating can be provided. This allows for the immediate interpretation of the quality of life for the individual at follow-up. As symptoms, and therefore the attendant bothersomeness, of incontinence diminish slowly, it is rather subjective as to whether its bothersomeness has actually improved. The ICIQ tool is a very effective means of collecting such data accurately.

Suggested standard statements

Below are examples of standard statements that you may wish to include in a pathway.

If patients are dry, itchy or sore in the vaginal or vulval area, consider oestrogen therapy (female patients).

Oestrogen supplementation improves the vaginal, urethral and trigonal epithelium and leads to restoration of pre-menopausal vaginal flora (Getliffe and Dolman, 2003). The vaginal epithelium may become inflamed, contributing to urinary symptoms such as frequency, urgency, dysuria, incontinence and/or recurrent infections. Moreover, it has been suggested that reduced oestrogen levels may affect periurethral tissues and contribute to pelvic laxity and stress incontinence. In association with hypoestrogenemia, changes in vaginal pH and vaginal flora may

Figure 5.2 Example of stress incontinence care pathway

Standard statement	Variance from standard statement and reason/comments
Visit 1	
Bothersome rating (ICIQ) this visit:	
Female patients: If patients are dry, itchy or sore in the vaginal or vulval area, consider oestrogen therapy.	
Stress incontinence information sheet given to female patients.	
Male patients: Information sheet for men datasheet.	
All patients: Stress incontinence information sheet discussed with patient; patient confirms they understand its content.	
Date and time of next visit agreed with patient (within 4–6 weeks).	
Visit 2	
Patient reviewed 4–6 weeks after Visit 1.	
Bothersome rating (ICIQ) this visit:	
If patient's symptoms have improved significantly, discharge.	
If symptoms not improved, continue CP.	

Patient says they have complied with the pelvic floor exercises and drinking advice; reinforce advice and continue with CP.	
Patient says they have not complied with PFEs and drinking advice; reinforce advice and continue CP.	
Date and time of next visit agreed with patient (within 4–6 weeks).	
Visit 3	
Patient reviewed within 4–6 weeks of Visit 2.	
Bothersome rating (ICIQ) this visit:	
If patient's symptoms have improved significantly, discharge.	
If patient's symptoms have not improved: refer to:	

TO BE COMPLETED BY ALL STAFF USING THE PATHWAY

Sign that you have met all standards or recorded variances for your part of the pathway

On discharge, sign and date

Full name	Designation	Initials	Sign	Date
Discharge date:		Signature:		

predispose post-menopausal women to urinary tract infection (UTI) (Castelo-Branco *et al.*, 2005). The authors found no evidence to support the prescription of oestrogen for women to alleviate stress incontinence without concurrent atrophic vaginitis. Therefore, oestrogen alone does not appear to be an effective treatment for urinary stress incontinence, but should be considered in the presence of urogenital atrophy. There are many conflicting studies on this and the reader is strongly recommended to consult the latest research.

Stress incontinence information sheet given to female patients.

Patients and/or carers have free access to evidenced-based information about bowel and bladder care that has been adapted to meet the individual patient's needs and/or those of their carer (Department of Health, 2003). There are guidelines on the importance of patient information, and a toolkit to help develop these can be downloaded from http://www.nhsidentity.nhs.uk/tools-and-resources/patient-information.

There is strong evidence to suggest that pelvic floor muscle exercises are effective in reducing the symptoms of stress urinary incontinence (Berghmans *et al.*, 1998).

Give out 'Information for men' datasheet (male patients).

Men may be taught pelvic floor exercises and should be given exercises that are specifically for them (Getliffe and Dolman, 2003)

Stress incontinence sheet discussed with patient. Patient confirms that they have understood its contents.

In order to elicit a contraction and for the patient to work maximally a careful explanation of what is expected should be given (Laycock and Haslam, 2002).

Date and time of next visit agreed with patient.

A trial of supervised pelvic floor muscle training of at least three months' duration should be offered as a first-line treatment to women with stress or mixed urinary incontinence (National Institute for Health and Clinical Excellence, 2006). The time spent on training will depend on the patient's problem and their response. Local resources will also dictate what follow-up may be, but it is always important when teaching exercises to see the patient regularly for support and advice.

Urge incontinence care pathway

Urgency, urge incontinence or an overactive bladder means having to pass urine because of a sudden desire to void and leaking before you reach the toilet. It is often associated with frequent visits to the toilet both day and night. The condition may arise as a result of gynaecological, urological, medical or even psychological pathology (Swami and Abrams, 1996).

Retraining the overactive bladder, along with advice about fluid intake, cutting down on caffeine, alcohol and fizzy drinks, is a first-line approach. After recording urinary frequency for a few days, targets are set by lengthening the time between each void, thus increasing bladder capacity. Pelvic floor exercises help to control the urge. In cases where leakage is occurring or holding is difficult drug therapy may be considered in the form of anticholinergics, which may be combined with electrostimulation. Figure 5.3 gives an example of an urgency care pathway.

Bothersome rating

Patients are asked their bothersome rating at each visit to check whether they are subjectively improving (Bayliss *et al.*, 2000a). The authors used a simple Likert scale. However, it is recommended that users consider using the ICIQ questionnaires discussed earlier in this chapter, as a specific score/rating can be provided. This allows for the immediate interpretation of the quality of life for the individual at follow-up. As symptoms, and therefore the attendant bothersomeness, of incontinence diminish slowly, it is rather subjective as to whether its bothersomeness has actually improved. The ICIQ tool is a very effective means of collecting such data accurately.

Figure 5.3 An example of an urgency care pathway

Standard statement	Variance from standard statement and reason/comments
Visit 1	
Bothersome rating (ICIQ) this visit:	
Female patients: If patients are dry, itchy, red or sore in the vaginal or vulval area, consider oestrogen therapy.	
All patients: If diagnosed with neurological dysfunction (e.g. MS, Parkinson's disease, diabetes, CVA), check for residual urine. If more than 100 ml, discuss with specialist clinician. If less, continue CP.	
Male patients: Give copy of information sheet for men.	
Female patients: Copy of information sheet for women given to patient.	
Information sheet discussed with patient; patient confirms they understand its contents.	
Patient given urinary journal and shown how to complete it.	
Date and time of next visit agreed with patient (within 4–6 weeks).	
Visit 2	
Bothersome rating (ICIQ) this visit:	
Patient reviewed within 4–6 weeks of Visit 1.	

Urinary journal reviewed with patient.	
If within 4–7 voids per day, fewer than two voids per night, continue with urge CP.	
If outside above parameters for voiding, refer to continence nurse specialist.	
'Urge' (pink) information sheet given at Visit 1 discussed and reinforced with patient.	
Date and time of next visit agreed with patient (within 4–6 weeks).	
Visit 3	
Patient reviewed within 4–6 weeks of Visit 2.	
Bothersome rating (ICIQ) this visit:	
Patient discharged if they feel they no longer have a problem or symptoms have improved significantly.	
If bothersome rating not improved, refer to:	

TO BE COMPLETED BY ALL STAFF USING THE PATHWAY

Sign that you have met all standards or recorded variances for your part of the pathway

On discharge sign and date

Full name	Designation	Initials	Sign	Date
Discharge date:		**Signature:**		

Suggested standard statements

Below are examples of standard statements that may be included in a pathway.

If patients are dry, itchy or sore in the vaginal or vulval area, consider oestrogen therapy (female patients).

See data for stress incontinence pathway (p. 75). However, one study (Moehrer *et al.*, 2003) did show an improvement for women with urgency of micturition. Overall, it was found that there were around one to two fewer voids within a 24-hour period amongst women treated with oestrogen. The effect again appeared to be larger amongst women with urge incontinence.

If diagnosed with neurological dysfunction (e.g. multiple sclerosis, Parkinson's disease, diabetes, CVA), check for residual urine. If more than 100 ml, discuss with clinical specialist. If less, continue care pathway.

The measurement of post-void residual volume by bladder scan or catheterisation should be performed if there are symptoms suggestive of voiding dysfunction or recurrent UTI (National Institute for Health and Clinical Excellence, 2006). If the amount retained is 100 ml or more, then some action should be taken (Getliffe and Dolman, 2003).

Urgency information sheet given to patient.

Patients and/or carers have free access to evidenced-based information about bowel and bladder care that has been adapted to meet individual patient needs and/or those of their carer (Department of Health, 2003).

Urgency information sheet discussed with patient; patient confirms that they understand its contents.

It is well recognised in the health care community that clear communication, the involvement of service users and the provision of timely, evidence-based information are key elements in moving towards a genuinely patient-centred service (National Institute for Health and Clinical Excellence, 2006).

Patient given urinary journal and shown how to complete it.

Bladder diaries are a reliable method of quantifying urinary frequency and incontinence episodes (National Institute for Health and Clinical Excellence, 2006). Bladder diaries should record frequency of micturition, volumes passed and information from the patient regarding circumstances surrounding any leaks. It could also include pad changes and fluid intake.

Date and time of next visit.

Bladder training for a minimum of six weeks should be offered as a first-line treatment to women with urge or mixed incontinence (National Institute for Health and Clinical Excellence, 2006). The time spent on training will depend on the patient's problem and their response. Local resources will also dictate what follow-up could be, but it is always important when teaching exercises or bladder training to see the patient regularly for support and advice. The bladder diary will need to be reviewed with the patient at the next visit and, if appropriate, intervals set for voiding.

Overflow incontinence care pathway

Overflow incontinence occurs when the bladder does not fully empty. It is characterised by difficulty in starting the urine flow, which is slow and may be intermittent. Urine builds up in the bladder, exceeding normal capacity, and frequent dribbling leakage can occur. This may be caused by an enlarged prostate in men forming an obstruction. Constipation may block the bladder outlet. Diseases, such as multiple sclerosis, CVA, Parkinson's disease or diabetes may affect nerves and stop the bladder from emptying properly. Obstruction and overflow can be caused in both men and women by urethral damage resulting in a stricture (Bardsley, 2000).

Enlargement of the prostate needs to be assessed. A digital rectal examination, laboratory investigation, prostate-specific antigen (PSA), symptom questionnaires, urine flow rate along with X-rays and ultrasound are all possibilities. From these results a management plan can be made. This may be surgical, medical or involve careful monitoring.

Figure 5.4   Example of an overflow care pathway

Standard statement	Variance from standard statement and reason/comments
Visit 1	
Bothersome rating (ICIQ) this visit:	
Patient given urinary journal and shown how to complete it.	
Male patients: Measure post-void residual urine. If more than 100 ml, refer to GP and/or continence service.	
Ask GP for prostate assessment.	
Give copy of 'For men only' information sheet.	
Female patients: Measure post-void residual urine. If more than 100 ml, refer to clinical specialist.	
If residual less than 100 ml, Information sheet given to patient.	
Information sheet discussed with patient; patient confirms they understand its contents.	
All patients: Date and time of next visit agreed with patient (within 2–4 weeks).	
Visit 2	
Bothersome rating (ICIQ) this visit:	
Patient reviewed within 2–4 weeks of Visit 1.	

Patient discharged if they feel they no longer have a problem or symptoms have improved significantly.	
If bothersome rating not improved and patient has not been referred for urological or other opinion, refer to:	

TO BE COMPLETED BY ALL STAFF USING THE PATHWAY

Sign that you have met all standards or recorded variances for your part of the pathway

On discharge sign and date

Full name	Designation	Initials	Sign	Date
Discharge date:		Signature:		

For patients who are not able to empty their bladder because of neurological disorders or a stricture, self-catheterisation may be required. If this is not possible, an in-dwelling catheter may be considered. Figure 5.4 gives an example of an overflow care pathway.

Bothersome rating

Patients are asked their bothersome rating at each visit to check whether they are subjectively improving (Bayliss *et al.*, 2000a). The authors used a simple Likert scale. However, it is recommended that users consider using the ICIQ questionnaires discussed earlier in this chapter, as a specific score/rating can be provided. This allows for immediate interpretation of the quality of life for the individual at follow-up. As symptoms, and therefore the attendant bothersomeness, of incontinence diminish slowly, it is rather subjective as to whether its bothersomeness has actually improved. The ICIQ tool is a very effective means of collecting such data accurately.

Suggested standard statements

Below are examples of standard statements that you may wish to include in a pathway.

Patient given urinary journal and shown how to complete it.

Bladder diaries are a reliable method of quantifying urinary frequency and incontinence episodes (National Institute for Health and Clinical Excellence, 2006).

Measure post-void residual urine. If more than 100 ml, refer to clinical specialist.

The measurement of post-void residual volume by bladder scan or catheterisation should be performed if there are symptoms suggestive of voiding dysfunction or recurrent UTI. If the amount retained is 100 ml or more, then some action should be taken (Getliffe and Dolman, 2003).

Perform prostate assessment (male patients).

Enlargement of the prostate through disease processes and age-associated changes can, owing to its position, serve to obstruct the outflow of urine (Getliffe and Dolman, 2003).

Give copy of information sheet for men.

There are some issues which are specific to male patients, and it is necessary therefore to have an information sheet designed that details these. For example, if a few drops of urine leak out after the patient has finished passing water, it may be that some urine is trapped in the outlet where the prostate used to be (Getliffe and Dolman, 2003).

Patient reviewed within 2–4 weeks of Visit 1.

If bothersome rating has not improved and patient has not been referred for urological or other opinions, refer to the continence service.

The use of these statements is recommended, and others can be added so long as the evidence base and/or best practice supports them. The preceding statements have been used to identify and treat the most common types of urinary incontinence. They are not exhaustive and are only provided to give both examples and guidelines to those who wish to design continence care pathways for their area of care.

Key summary points

- A Symptom Profile will identify the type of incontinence.
- Many different pathways can be designed by patient groups.
- Stress, urge and overflow are the most frequently occurring types of incontinence.
- Standard statements should not deviate from the evidence base.

Chapter 6

Bowel care pathway

This chapter considers the design and impact that care pathways may have on bowel care. It looks at the possible standard statements that may be employed and the rationale and criteria for them. It also defines the various signs and symptoms and provides the evidence to underpin the use of these with care pathways.

It is important that users of the pathway and patients have a basic understanding of the physiology of the bowel and an understanding of what normal control of defecation actually is. This is necessary because they must be able to understand and comprehend what is being asked of them. For example, patients may mistreat symptoms of perceived constipation with strong laxatives, or increase insoluble fibre in their diet with no commensurate increase in fluid intake. The physiology of the bowel is explained here in detail in order that information sheets can be tailored to the specific patient cohort.

Physiology of the bowel

When faeces enter the rectum, their presence is detected by sensory nerve endings. These are found in the muscles around the rectum. This results in a sensation of rectal fullness and the desire to defecate. The mechanics of defecation involve the relaxation of the external and internal sphincters. The internal anal sphincter is under autonomic control and the external anal sphincter is under both autonomic and voluntary control. Approximately

150 ml of faeces cause autonomic relaxation of the anal sphincter. Faeces then enter the anal canal and sensitive nerve endings relay messages to the brain, which are interpreted as urgency. Sensitive squamous epithelium can distinguish between flatus, fluid and stool entering the anal canal, even if the person is asleep.

If it is convenient to defecate, the external sphincter relaxes. A reflex action from the spinal cord will initiate the emptying of the bowel. This action can be inhibited by the cerebral cortex. Therefore, if defecation is inconvenient, the process may be delayed, thereby giving the patient control over this mechanism. The stool is then passed by muscular contraction. The position of the person is also important, as gravity and the abdominal effort (straining) aid expulsion. Unless the stool is hard owing to constipation, only a small amount of abdominal effort is required to propel the stool through the anal canal. Any injury or disease, which interferes with this mechanism, for example pelvic floor damage following childbirth, can result in constipation. It is important that any pathway information pack contains this information, plus information about the functions of the bowel (Box 6.1).

Box 6.1 Function of the bowel

1. **Storage:** The colon stores unabsorbed food residue. Within 72 hours of intake, 70% of food residue has been excreted. The remaining 30% stays in the colon for up to a week or more. The longer food residue remains in the colon, the more water is reabsorbed and the stools produced are harder.
2. **Absorption:** Sodium, water, chloride and some fat-soluble vitamins are absorbed from the colon. Some drugs, e.g. some steroids and aspirin, are also absorbed by the colonic membrane.
3. **Secretion:** Mucus is secreted by the colon to lubricate the faeces and aid expulsion.
4. **Synthesis of some vitamins:** Bacteria which colonise the colon are responsible for the production of small amounts of vitamin K, thiamine, folic acid and riboflavin.
5. **Elimination:** The main function of the colon is the propulsion of the faecal matter and absorption of fluid.

Suggested standard statements

Suggested standard statements that you may wish to include in a bowel care pathway (Figure 6.1):

If the patient has any signs of undiagnosed rectal bleeding or black tarry stools and is not taking ferrous sulphate, stop the pathway and refer to doctor immediately.

Rectal bleeding is the passage of blood from the anus. It is an abnormal event that may occur at any time during the human life cycle. Although often attributed to the presence of benign anorectal conditions, the presence of neoplastic disease must be excluded (Helfand *et al.*, 1997, in Norton and Chelvanayagam, 2004).

The presence of fresh blood in the faeces should immediately alert the health care professional to the risk of rectal or bowel tumour. However, other causes may be:

- haemorrhoids and anal fissure
- inflammatory bowel disease such as ulcerative colitis
- solitary rectal ulcer syndrome, benign ulcers caused by chronic constipation and straining
- diverticulitis/diverticular disease.

The patient may well have a previous diagnosis of one of these. It is very important to establish what this diagnosis was and when it was made and by whom. Ferrous sulphate can mimic the sight of digested blood and black tarry stool and a possible pathology higher in the bowel must also be excluded.

Using the obstruction checklist, observe the patient for signs and symptoms of obstruction. If present, stop pathway and refer to doctor immediately.

Intestinal obstruction is a blockage of the small intestine or the colon that prevents food or fluid passing through. Signs and symptoms may include:

- nausea
- vomiting
- constipation and ability to pass flatus

Figure 6.1 An example of a bowel care pathway

Full name:		Date of birth:
Address:		Postcode:
		Tel:
GP:	Practice:	NHS NO.
Assessor:	Designation:	Tel:

What has been the effect of your bowel problem on your life?

How much does it bother you? (Tick your choice or give ICIQ score.)

....

a lot ☐   *moderately* ☐   *a little* ☐   *not at all* ☐

What is your normal bowel habit?

How do you maintain this?

Standard statement	Variance from standard statement and reason/comments
If the patient has any signs of undiagnosed bleeding or black tarry stool and is not taking ferrous sulphate, stop pathway and refer to clinician immediately.	
Patient drinks .... amount of fluid per day.	
If patient drinks volumes outside parameters of fluid template, advise them to drink appropriate amount.	
If patient is taking medication from the list provided, consider review.	
Establish constipation using signs and symptoms chart and record findings.	
Report any abnormal changes in bowel habit.	
If faecal incontinence, use algorithm.	
Use fibre scoring chart to establish fibre levels. If 12 or fewer, give information sheet and advice on increasing fibre in diet.	

Standard statement	Variance from standard statement and reason/comments
If patient unable or unwilling to comply, consider fibre supplements.	
If patient is in discomfort, consider abdominal massage technique.	
Administer and record appropriate treatment.	
Obtain patient's consent to any invasive procedure.	
Establish follow-up procedure.	

TO BE COMPLETED BY ALL STAFF USING THE PATHWAY

Sign to confirm that you have met all standards or recorded variances

Full name	Designation	Initials	Sign	Date

- abdominal distension, more common in large bowel obstruction
- abdominal tenderness
- diarrhoea
- history of infrequent bowel movement.

In small bowel obstruction the pain tends to be colicky, cramping and intermittent in nature, with spasms lasting a few minutes. The pain tends to be central and mid-abdominal. Vomiting tends to occur before constipation. In large bowel obstruction the pain is felt in the lower abdomen and the spasms last longer. Constipation occurs earlier and vomiting may be less prominent.

Causes of small bowel obstruction include:

- adhesions from previous abdominal surgery
- hernias containing bowel
- Crohn's disease, causing adhesions or inflammatory strictures
- neoplasms, benign or malignant
- intussusception in children
- volvulus
- ischaemic strictures
- foreign bodies (e.g. gallstones or swallowed objects).

Causes of large bowel obstruction may include:

- neoplasm
- hernias
- inflammatory bowel disease
- colonic volvulus (sigmoid, caecal, transverse colon)
- faecal impaction
- colon atresia
- benign strictures (diverticular disease).

If patient's fluid intake is less than 1.5 litres per day, recommend this as a minimum.

This is the recommended volume (National Institute for Health and Clinical Excellence, 2007) to prevent constipation.

If patient is taking medication from the list provided, consider review.

Medication can be a significant cause of constipation. Ginsberg *et al.* (2007) note that 60% of drugs listed in the *Physicians' Desk Reference* gave constipation as an adverse effect. Most drugs that cause constipation directly or indirectly interfere with the physiology of colonic transit. It is possible that an alternative medication may be prescribed or that a suitable laxative be prescribed or recommended alongside the constipation causing medication.

Although a list of medications is provided in Appendix 2, it is strongly recommended that the list be used only as a basis for a care pathway. Primarily, this is because the list must be regularly updated and, secondly, because if a pathway is being written for a diagnostic related group of patients, then the list of medication which pertains to that group should be considered in greater detail by the multidisciplinary team. It may well be that these pathways could include prescribing recommendations.

Establish constipation using signs and symptoms chart and record findings.

Constipation is merely a symptom, not a disease. It reflects either slowed colonic transit and/or impairment (Thompson *et al.*, 1999). Its impact may vary from slight, causing no disruption of life, to

Box 6.2 Standard diagnostic criteria for functional incontinence

At least 12 weeks, which need not be consecutive, in the preceding 12 months if more than two of the following symptoms are detected in an adult:

- fewer than three bowel movements per week
- straining during > 25% of defecations
- lumpy or hard stools in > 25% of defecations
- sensation of incomplete evacuation in > 25% of defecations
- sensation of anorectal obstruction or blockade in > 25% of defecations
- manual manoeuvres to facilitate > 25% of defecations
- loose stools are not present, and there are insufficient criteria for
- irritable bowel syndrome

Source: Thompson *et al.*, 1999.

severe, when the patient's social and personal functioning is grossly disrupted (Norton and Chelvanayagam, 2004).

In simple terms constipation is when a person passes faeces less often or finds it difficult to pass a stool. It is relevant here to give the Rome II Diagnostic criteria for chronic constipation in more detail. For the recommended standard diagnostic criteria for functional incontinence see Box 6.2.

The criteria are fewer than three bowel movements per week and at least two of the above symptoms met to validate the diagnosis.

Constipation has already been discussed in Chapter 4, where diet, mobility and environmental factors are covered in detail. Other causes of constipation include:

- dehydration causing hard stools. Faeces need to be large enough to stimulate gut contraction and soft enough to pass easily along the gut.
- lack of dietary fibre. This reduces the weight and bulk of stools.
- ignoring the call to stool. This may be because people want to avoid using public toilets or are too busy. Water then continues to be absorbed and the faeces become harder and more difficult to pass. It can also result in changes to how the bowel works.
- immobility. This is a particular cause in older patients but can also affect those who have suffered a cerebral vascular accident,

spinal cord injury or have a neurological disease such as multiple sclerosis. Increasing physical activity as part of rehabilitation may help.

■ third- or fourth-degree tear during delivery.
■ metabolic or endocrine diseases such as hypothyroidism, hyperthyroidism, diabetes mellitus and Addison's disease.
■ neurological, including spinal cord lesions and peripheral lesions leading to neuropathy.
■ medications. These can slow peristalsis and increase transit times such as opioids (e.g. codeine, tricyclic antidepressants and iron). Diuretics may cause the stool to become drier.
■ severe illness, surgery or chronic illness.
■ those relating to the colon, which include constriction of the intestine, which may be caused by strictures, diverticula or tumours.
■ rectal problems, such as rectal prolapse or rectocele.
■ painful conditions, such as an anal fissure or an anal sphincter injury.
■ haemorrhoids.

Signs and symptoms of constipation vary from patient to patient but may include some of the following:

■ A change in bowel habit or stool frequency, resulting in less frequent bowel actions.
■ A change in stool consistency, resulting in dry and hard stools.
■ Bulky stools that are difficult and painful to pass.
■ Straining to pass a stool.
■ A feeling of incomplete emptying after bowel evacuation.
■ A history of laxative use.
■ Abdominal bloating and pain.
■ Lethargy, nausea, headaches, loss of appetite, halitosis.

It is essential that the first-level assessment includes a bowel habit diary and a one-week recording of dietary intake. These two records form the basis for making a diagnosis (Getliffe and Dolman, 2003). Information should include frequency of defecation, type of stool and episodes of incontinence as a minimum. Depending on the patient group, other signs and symptoms may be recorded as described above. Neurologically impaired patients may have pelvic floor uncoordination and an increased threshold of rectal sensation (Weisel *et al.*, 2000).

It may also be helpful to provide information about correct positioning for defecation, which includes advising patients to sit with feet supported on a stool using the brace and lift techniques as described by Norton and Chelvanayagam (2004).

Report any abnormal changes in bowel habit.

Changes in bowel habit may indicate the presence of a neoplasm. This must be excluded before any therapy is initiated. A change in bowel habit includes any constant change in bowel frequency, colour, consistency or shape of stools.

Use a fibre scoring chart to establish fibre levels. If less than 30 g per day, give information sheet and advice on increasing dietary fibre.

Fibre has been shown to increase the weight and bulkiness of stools, thereby aiding defecation (Getliffe and Dolman, 2003). The introduction of fibre into the diet should be gradual to avoid discomfort or bloating. It is also important to increase fluid intake, especially in older patients, to avoid dehydration.

There are two types of dietary fibre: soluble and insoluble. Soluble fibre is broken down by enzyme-producing bacteria present in the colon to produce energy and gas and bulky stools. This fibre forms a gel-like substance which can bind to other substances in the gut. It also has the extra benefits of lowering cholesterol levels and slowing down the entry of glucose into the blood, thereby improving blood sugar control.

Foods predominantly high in insoluble fibre are:

■ fruit and vegetables with their skins and pips
■ wholegrain cereals (wheat, rye, rice)
■ nuts and some pulses.

Insoluble fibre is less easily broken down by bacteria in the colon, but holds water very effectively (up to 15 times its weight in water) thus contributing to an increase in stool weight. It is this fibre that is often referred to as *nature's broom* and is thought to have many protective effects on the gut. It should be noted that raising fibre may provoke abdominal distension and flatulence in patients with slow transit constipation. A patient information sheet providing data on fibre content can help people to make suitable adjustments to their diet. A diet diary can also help to identify normal routines, likes and dislikes and enables the health care professional to make suggestions for alternatives.

If the patient is unable or unwilling to comply, consider fibre supplements.

Bulk-forming agents consist of natural (ispaghula or psyllium) or synthetic polysaccharides or cellulose derivatives (methylcellulose) that act in a manner similar to dietary fibre. The agents absorb water and expand to fill the colon with soft, non-absorbable residue and appear to have few side effects. Caution is advised in using bulking agents in older patients as this may lead to severe dehydration.

If patient is in discomfort, consider abdominal massage technique.

Abdominal massage as a therapy to relieve constipation has been known to be effective for many hundreds of years, but was given a higher profile in the 1870s by the American John Kellogg (inventor of cornflakes). He recommended 'abdominal massage with a leather-coated cannonball weighing three to four pounds for men with sluggish colons'.

Slow massage relieves muscle tension, thereby improving blood circulation and lymphatic drainage. It may also alleviate constipation or reduce the need for medication (Getliffe and Dolman, 2003). Ayas *et al.* (2006) report that abdominal massage has positive effects on some clinical aspects of neurological bowel dysfunction, increasing the number of bowel movements per week and decreasing the total colonic transit time.

The aim of the massage is to release spasm in the abdomen to allow normal gut activity and increase peristalsis (Resende *et al.*, 1993). It may be especially useful in patients who are hemiplegics or paraplegic, as exercise may not be possible. It should also be avoided in patients with abdominal hernias or those who have recently undergone abdominal surgery.

Records results of digital rectal examination.

Digital rectal examination can assess anal sphincter tone reasonably well. Easy finger insertion with gaping of the anus on finger removal indicates poor internal sphincter tone, while reduced squeeze pressure around the finger when asking the patient to 'squeeze and pull up' suggests external sphincter weakness. A rectal examination is also essential for identifying stool impaction (Norton and Chelvanayagam, 2006).

Digital rectal examination establishes:

- the presence or absence of faeces in the rectum; the amount and consistency in order to assess for faecal loading and consistency of stool
- anal tone, both resting and under voluntary contraction in those patients with bowel dysfunction associated with lax pelvic muscle tone or faecal incontinence.

Digital rectal examination is not a reliable indicator of constipation as the colon may be faecal loaded higher. It is recommended that all incontinent patients without rectal stool impaction undergo plain abdominal X-ray to establish or rule out the diagnosis of overflow (Norton and Chelvanayagam, 2006).

Document consent for digital rectal examination.

It is important that informed written or verbal consent is given prior to a digital rectal examination or before a manual evacuation of faeces is carried out. A consent form must be used and a copy of this must be kept in the patient's records. A note must also be made in the care plan and signed by the patient and the registered nurse. Local consent policies must be taken into account when writing a statement about this for the pathway.

If the patient is cognitively impaired, the decision must be made by the medical practitioner involved in the patient's care, who must sign with the patient's nursing team leader that this course of action has been entered into and is appropriate for the patient (Addison and Smith, 1995). The reader is directed to the Royal College of Nursing's guidance for nurses *Bowel Care Including Digital Rectal Examination and the Manual Removal of Faeces* (2008) for further information.

Many Trusts now offer training in digital rectal examination and manual evacuation of faeces, and if these are available they should form part of the pathway, to ensure that only suitably skilled staff carry out these procedures.

At this point it may be relevant to include in the pathway the administration of medication. It is not intended here to rehearse in detail data about medication, as this will depend entirely on the patient group which the pathway is intended for and the local formulary and advice.

Consider the possibility of autonomic dysreflexia.

Care needs to be taken to check whether the patient has a history of any autonomic dysreflexia before undertaking any investigation or procedure that could precipitate such an event, and expert advice should be sought if necessary.

Autonomic dysreflexia is a potentially life-threatening problem seen particularly in patients with cervical injuries above the sympathetic outflow but may also occur in those with high thoracic lesions above T6. It may occur at any time after the period of spinal shock and is most commonly caused by a distended bladder but may also be caused by other conditions which cause visceral stimulation, for example infection, loaded colon or anal fissure.

The effect is that there is reflex sympathetic overactivity below the level of the spinal cord lesion, causing vasoconstriction and systemic hypertension. The carotid and aortic baroreceptors are stimulated and respond via the vasomotor centre with increased vagal tone and resulting bradycardia; but peripheral vasodilation that would normally have relieved the hypertension does not occur, as stimuli cannot pass distally through the injured cord.

Symptoms of autonomic dysreflexia are, characteristically, pounding headache, profuse sweating, flushing or blotchiness above the level of the lesion (see Box 6.3). Without prompt treatment intercranial haemorrhage may occur (Grundy and Swain, 1996).

Treatment consists of removing the precipitating cause. It may also affect patients with an injury at T6–T10.

Box 6.3 Signs and symptoms of autonomic dysreflexia

- Severe headache with blurred vision and dizziness
- Restlessness and anxiety
- Change in heart rate
- Profuse sweating
- Flushing above the level of the spinal cord injury

Consider the use of bowel movement stimulation.

Many individuals with a spinal injury are able to control bowel movements by stimulating the anus with a finger. This causes a reflex emptying of the rectum.

Digital stimulation may be achieved either by inserting suppositories or by inserting a gloved finger just inside the anus. Gentle rotation of the finger may stimulate the rectum to contract (Royal College of Nursing, 2008).

Standard statements used in bowel care will depend on the speciality that the pathway is being implemented in, and to what level and competency care is provided. For example, a pathway designed for use in a spinal injuries unit must include statements on autonomic dysreflexia, whilst a pathway designed for use with older patients would not warrant this. A single pathway may be sufficient; however, in situations where more complex care is to be provided, it may be necessary to write more pathways. It may also be helpful to provide an algorithm as part of the pathway for faecal incontinence such as the one shown below as Figure 6.2.

There are many causes of faecal incontinence, including anal sphincter/pelvic floor damage or pathology, neurological dysfunction (including cognitive dysfunction) and faecal impaction with overflow. However, it is essential that the cause of the faecal incontinence is established prior to any advice or treatment, and therefore it may be helpful to provide an algorithm as part of the pathway for faecal incontinence, such as the one shown in Figure 6.2.

Algorithms cannot take the place of a pathway as there is no variance tracking mechanism attached; however, it could be possible to design a tracking system to run alongside. Care must be taken to ensure that all users are aware of such a system and that it is easily accessible and easy to use.

A useful pathway could encompass faecal incontinence that has a diagnosis of anal sphincter/pelvic floor damage and would vary according to the level of competence and resources locally available. Anal sphincter exercises should be included but the pathway could also include criteria for biofeedback, if the service were available. A section on the provision of products to manage the incontinence should be included, as should the provision of advice on skin care.

At the beginning of the chapter it was stated that it is important that all users of the pathway have an understanding of the functions of the bowel. It is equally important that they are able to pass some

Figure 6.2 Faecal incontinence algorithm

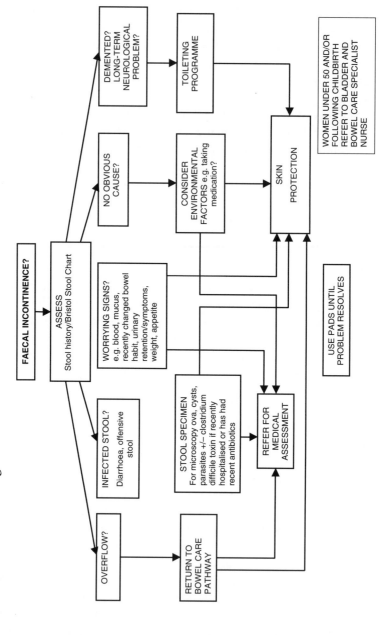

of this information to the patient. Common problems can occur when patients increase insoluble fibre consumption with no commensurate increase in fluid intake. Suggested patient information sheets are contained in the appendices (pp. 137–184) together with information sheets, which may be used by staff or for teaching.

Key summary points

- It is important to understand the physiology of defecation.
- Specific information sheets should be tailored to the patient cohort.
- Dietary manipulation can be effective in curing constipation.
- Nurses must be competent to undertake digital rectal examination.
- Specific pathways should be considered by diagnostic group.
- Algorithms may be used but must have variance tracking systems attached.

Chapter 7

Involving patients and other experts

Involvement of users

When referring to *users* of pathways, primarily we mean patients of continence care services that are using, or intend to use, pathways. In the literature *user involvement* has two meanings. The term can be used to mean the user involvement in organising health services and also mean the organisation of health services around the user, that is patient-centred health services (Clarke *et al.*, 2004). The use of care pathways is a way of organising health services around the user, as is the Expert Patients Programme (detailed below). In this book both meanings of the term user involvement are adopted, as patients have been involved in the development of pathways and the validation of these documents.

Involving users in planning and service delivery improves services by making them more responsive. In this sense user involvement can be seen as a type of accountability to the patient. Perhaps less frequently cited reasons for involving users are to:

- ensure confidence in health services
- understand patient expectations
- shape service provider perspectives
- shape priorities for service or to develop solutions (Smith and Ross 2004).

All health services have been required to consult and involve patients and the public (Department of Health, 1999). There are,
for example, the surveys to monitor NHS performance from the
patient's perspective, named the *NHS Patient Survey Programme*
(Department of Health, 2003). *The NHS in England: the operating
framework for 2007/08* talks about patient choice providing 'a powerful incentive for providers to respond to patients' preferences,
driving up quality and improving access to services' (Department
of Health, 2006).

> *As well as becoming more responsive to the patients who use it, the NHS
> needs to be more accountable to the citizens who fund it. There are a
> number of requirements aimed at ensuring a greater connection between
> PCTs and their communities, and that, as well as choice, citizens have
> more 'voice' in the healthcare system, particularly where this is not often
> heard, for example in public health/prevention. (Department of Health,
> 2006)*

This same document sets out potential benefits for patients and
carers as:

- Better-quality services that are more responsive to the needs of
  patients, leading to better outcomes of care and improvements
  in health and well-being.
- Policy and planning decisions that are more patient-focused.
- Improved communications between organisations and the com-
  munities they serve.
- Greater ownership of local health services, and a stronger understanding of why and how they need to change and develop.

User involvement should be seen in the context of wider involvement of the public in the NHS. To reflect this emphasis, the
Department of Health funds a national advisory Group, Involve
(http://www.invo.org.uk/), that is intended 'to promote and support active public involvement in NHS, public health and social
care research'.

This chapter looks at the ways in which patients as users have
been involved in the development of continence care pathways as
well as other ways they could potentially be involved. It outlines
the process of involvement, discussing who to include, how and at

what point to include users. For our purposes nurses are also users of the pathways, as are carers of patients with incontinence.

This chapter is based on the authors' knowledge of successfully applying research skills and on existing studies in the literature. Also brought to the book are the means by which users have been involved in the development of pathways, including:

- an audit of nurses who had received copies of the pathways, asking for their experiences of the application of pathways
- validation of the content of the continence care pathways paperwork by health care professionals
- a focus group with users and carers of continence services in Swindon to evaluate the continence care service and validate the information sheets and pathways documentation.

This chapter endeavours to equip the reader with the skills to carry out their own audits and to enable them to involve users in the process mapping and/or local adaption of care pathways.

The mind map in Figure 7.1 captures the headlines of the various elements of the involvement of users in the process of the development of care pathways. This chapter follows this mind map by expanding on the points made in the six points on the map.

What is patient involvement?

Involvement of patients can take various forms. It can be part of the process mapping and local adoption of pathways which were outlined in the Chapter 3. The patient can be involved in identifying the steps of the patient's journey through the continence services and their views on the efficiency and effectiveness of the process, including administrative, to feed into an improved service design.

Most of this chapter is dedicated to detailing how users can be involved in the process of development and adoption of pathways. The involvement of users relevant to patients and staff within the field of continence care can take other forms, two of which are outlined first in this chapter, namely the Expert Patient Programme and user groups.

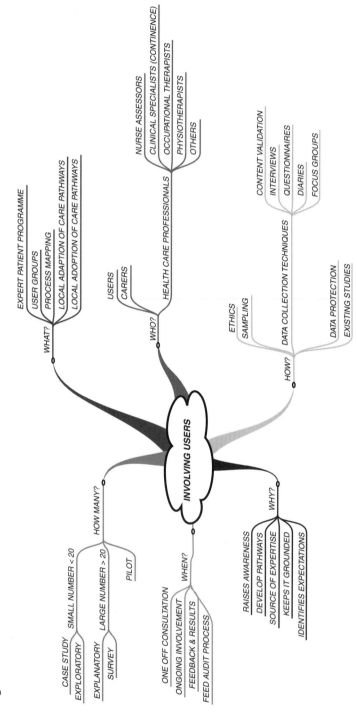

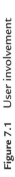

Figure 7.1 User involvement

The Expert Patients Programme

The Expert Patients Programme is a lay-led self-management programme that has been specifically developed for people living with long-term conditions. The aim of the programme is to support people to increase their confidence, improve their quality of life and better manage their condition. (Department of Health website, http://www.dh.gov.uk/en/Aboutus/ MinistersandDepartmentLeaders/ChiefMedicalOfficer/ProgressOnPolicy/ ProgressBrowsableDocument/DH_4102757)

The Expert Patients Programme is designed to include chronic conditions which include elements to help and support those issues that cause embarrassment, like incontinence. To help provide help to carers, the Expert Patients Programme has also developed a course called 'Looking after me', which tackles some of the issues carers face.

The Expert Patients Programme is based on previous projects, including the Living with Long-term Illness Project and the Living Well Project in this country and a model of care developed at Stanford University in California, where patients are encouraged to take control over living with a chronic condition. It is not the only current such project; for example, there is the DAFNE (Dose Adjustment for Normal Eating) Programme that adjusts insulin doses to fit with people's lifestyles.

On the Expert Patients Programme individuals living with long-term problems attend expert courses (which are made up of six sessions, each lasting two and a half hours per week) that are led by people who have a long-term condition themselves. They develop skills and techniques that would mean they could take over managing their conditions, helping them to solve problems, plan for the future and think more positively about themselves. The programme has been described as a 'revolution' that patients are more 'expert' than their doctor in the management of their condition (BBC Radio 4, 2005). However, older patients may be used to a more paternal approach to medicine rather than the patient-centred care that this programme is based on.

The pilots were successfully run from 2002 to 2004 and the programme was centrally managed by the Department of Health and implemented by the Primary Care Trusts. More recently, the White Paper *Our Health, Our Care, Our Say: A New Direction for Community Services*, made a commitment to establish a new community interest company to market and deliver the Expert Patients Programme (Department of Health, 2006a).

Internal evaluation data from approximately 1 000 Expert Patients Programme participants, who completed the course between January 2003 and January 2005, indicate that the programme is achieving improved health outcomes for patients and is reducing the degree to which they use health care services. Patients feel more confident and symptoms are less severe. Patients feel better prepared to get more out of health services.

Independent evaluation of the Expert Patients Programme has also been carried out by a national team of researchers based at the National Primary Care Research and Development Centre (NPCRDC) of the University of Manchester and the NPCRDC of the Centre for Health Economics at the University of York (Rogers *et al.*, 2006).

User groups

One type of user group is a *critical friends group*. This begins with a review, in the form of a questionnaire to users, of service provision. Users are asked to assess how well the service is performing, and as such are involved in a process mapping exercise. The focus group in Swindon, made up of carers and users, that the authors were involved with was set up to make this assessment (see below). Critical friends groups go a step further, though: when the data are gathered, a few users are asked to meet with staff – a critical friends group – to discuss the findings and help identify future priorities for the service and possible solutions.

The *Improvement leaders' guide* entitled *Involving Patients and Carers* published by the NHS Institute for Innovation and Improvement (2005a) uses the example of a GP practice administering and collecting the results from an Improving Practice Questionnaire. Once the data are collected, a few patients are asked to come to the practice and talk about the results, together with staff from the practice. Areas for improvement are identified and prioritised, and solutions planned.

There are groups that provide support for carers (as users). For example, one of the authors had contact with the Swindon Carers Centre (http://www.carers.org/local/south-west/swindon/), which provides advice and social support to carers in the Swindon area.

This group was a very useful contact in helping set up the focus group in Swindon with users and carers.

Of course, being able to set up and, equally importantly, maintain such user groups relies on resources being available.

Who to involve

Anyone who is, or will be, involved in the use of pathways either as staff or as users and carers can be involved. This chapter has already mentioned users and carers, but there are also health care professionals who carry out continence assessments or give continence advice. This group may include nurse assessors, clinical specialists, occupational therapists and physiotherapists.

The authors involved users and carers in a focus group event to find out their views of a continence service. They also carried out a survey of nurses that use pathways as part of the development of pathways to find out their experiences of using pathways. Both these items are detailed below.

When to involve users

Involvement can be one-off, like a focus group or a content validation exercise, such as the authors have been involved with in developing and applying the continence care pathways. These are described below. Other means of involving users, for example conducting interviews and encouraging them to keep diaries, are also described in the **How to involve users** section below.

User involvement in the development of care pathways could be ongoing, in the form of user groups. Whether this is possible depends on what resources are available for such groups to be established and then to receive ongoing support.

There is a need to involve users in feedback and results. Smith and Ross found that in their review of the cataract care pathways literature 'there is a clear deficit . . . . with regard to incorporating patient experiences into the progressive development of services' (Smith and Ross, 2004). With the development of care pathways it was intended that this deficit be avoided by including patients in the development and validation of the pathways themselves. Also users' views were to be included in the ongoing development of the pathways by exploiting variance tracking to the full.

How many users?

How many users to involve depends on the type of information and input that is required from users, in other words the answer to *how many* will depend on why the involvement is being done. If health care professionals wish to prompt in-depth, detailed responses from users, a good number of respondents to have would be around about ten. If the aim is to cover issues in less detail but more broadly, then greater numbers of users will be involved. Such a study will involve at least fifty participants. For example, the authors' questionnaire survey of nurses' experiences of the use of pathways was completed by 144 (Bayliss *et al.*, 2003).

How to involve users

Consideration needs to be given to the ethics of the involvement of users, sampling and data protection issues.

Any involvement of users in audit or research requires consideration to the ethical aspects of what is proposed. This means making sure the study is carried out properly and there are no attempts to involve participants without their knowledge or mislead them about the true nature of the study. The research will need to adhere to the recent Mental Capacity Act 2005, which covers research with people that lack the capacity to consent to the research. There are Research Ethic Committees (RECs) from which permission for the involvement of patients and staff needs to be sought. The National Patient Safety Agency's National Research Ethics Service website will help identify a local REC (http://www.nres.npsa.nhs.uk/contacts/find-your-local-rec/). Some of the questions that need addressing are:

- Do individuals have the right not to take part?
- Are they fully informed about the true nature of the study?
- Do they know what they are letting themselves in for?

In practice consent is sought from the user before taking part in the study, usually by both parties signing a consent form, the user having read and understood an information sheet about the study. It needs to be made clear in this paperwork that users can withdraw from the study at any time.

Sampling or selecting which users to include needs to be done objectively, and without bias. This is one way to ensure that what we have found to be true in a particular situation and at a particular time can be applied more generally. In picking users it is inappropriate to select favoured patients. Neither can the whole population be consulted, which is where the sampling comes in, that is a sample is a selection from the population. In selecting the patients for a focus group with users and carers in Swindon the authors took a cross section of the total service user population picked along the lines of age, symptoms, treatment and gender in order that the sample was generally representative of service users.

Any information about users that the researcher has and holds needs to be kept safe and conform to the Data Protection Act 1998. In practice completely anonymising all data held, including personal details and users' recorded responses (either written or oral), will resolve this issue. An ethics committee, to which an application for approval of involvement of users may be sought, will require reassurance that users' personal data will be safely stored.

When a health care professional seeks the involvement of users to help with research, whether to explore the views of certain patient cohorts in detail or to survey the general population more broadly, they must establish a means of collecting the information. A study that reviewed research on behalf of the Commission for Healthcare Improvement (known then as the CHI, and now as the Healthcare Commission) on patient experiences of care pathways in three areas (cataract, hip replacement and knee arthroscopy) identified the methods through which patients had been asked about their experiences in existing studies (Smith and Ross, 2004). Different techniques used include questionnaires, content validation, focus groups, patient shadowing, patient diaries, interviews and critical friends groups. The authors have used some of these methods and here we will go on to describe our studies, methods used and findings. The chapter ends with a brief outline of other techniques in a section on how to involve users locally.

Whatever data-collection technique is employed to involve users, there should be a pilot, or dummy run. This can be undertaken with a small group of respondents before the main study to see whether questions work and gauge whether the information that is received will answer the questions that the study seeks to address.

Questionnaires

Questionnaires work best with standardized questions, where the questions mean the same thing to different respondents. They are best for descriptive purposes, and postal or self-administered questionnaires have the advantage of being efficient at providing large amounts of data, at relatively low cost, in a short period of time. They allow anonymity, which can encourage frankness when sensitive areas like incontinence are involved. They can be self-administered or administered by an interviewer. Unfortunately self-administered surveys can have a low response rate and as the characteristics of non-respondents are unknown it is therefore not possible to say whether they are representative. A common question concerns what is an acceptable response rate. There is no right answer here, but above 50% is acceptable. The response rate in the authors' study of nurses' experiences of the use of pathways was 51%. The questionnaire was sent to the nurses who had received copies of the pathways in the three years prior to the audit in 2002. The survey was conducted as an audit as to nurses' experiences of using the pathways and as such was part of the process of developing the pathways (Bayliss et al., 2003).

The questionnaire asked about use of the care pathways and the nature of any changes that had been made. The audit found that 43% (n = 32) of respondents were currently using the care pathways. Care pathways were felt to be an effective method of assessing continence and providing an equitable quality of care for the patients. Moreover, some respondents had gone on to write pathways for other areas, for example children, intermittent self-catheterisations, residential/nursing home residents etc. Of those that were not using them, the most common reasons were insufficient resources (n = 18) and lack of capacity to train staff (n = 35). The original pathways had been changed by 26 of the 32 respondents currently using them within their organisations. Changes had been made primarily to the generic assessment pathway, followed by the specific pathways for stress, urgency and overflow. The main reason for the changes were to make the pathways easier to use (n = 24), but also to fit in with local practice (n = 11). Local resource issues (n = 80) were also given as reasons for alterations. Some changes had been made to get round resource issues, such as coding with symbols as no colour printing was available. It was disappointing to note that so few changes had been made as a result of variance tracking as this system is the backbone of care pathways. Variance tracking should be the most frequently used change agent for care pathways. Without regular revisions of care pathways, taking into account all the deviations or variances from the anticipated care, care pathways are no longer dynamic; instead, they become out-of-date lists of prescribed care, which do not take into account local needs or issues. This was addressed as part of an information pack which was produced as a result of the audit and at a subsequent conference.

Content validation

This section sets out the means by which the pathways were validated. It describes the processes involved and continues by setting out how this process of validation added value to the pathways, with examples of modifications and feedback. It also outlines how validation can be undertaken locally. This discussion is appropriate in the context of a growing trend to ask patients about the accessibility and format of patient information. This is discussed by Coulter *et al.* (1998) and Duman (2003). The Health Services Research Unit at the University of Aberdeen published *Producing Information about Health and Health Care Interventions: A practical guide* (O'Donnell and Entwistle, 2003).

Two methods were used to validate our continence care pathways: content validation using health care professionals to validate the content of the pathways and a focus group of patients to improve the continence care service. These methods of checking the pathways are set out in the sections that follow. The feedback that these methods generated was then used to make changes to the pathways and reflects the dynamic nature of these documents.

The design of the pathways was based on scientific research in the field of continence care. Extensive literature searches of existing research generated specific items within the pathways as well as the overall emphasis of the pathways. Although the information contained in the care pathways was entirely evidence-based, it had never been presented before in a manner which would provide diagnosis and treatment to those nurses who may not have the requisite continence skills to make such judgements. It was necessary to find a way to ensure that the care pathways would be effective in practice and that they were relevant to practice. A method of content validation is described by Lynn (1986), where the validation process is carried out as a means of checking what was produced, by using experts (in this instance practising professionals in continence care). This determines the content representativeness and relevance of the items of an instrument by the application of a judgement process. How this was applied is set out in Bayliss *et al.* (2001).

The expert sample was selected by the continence care pathways development group on the basis of their expertise in the continence field. Lynn (1986) comments that a minimum number of five experts is necessary to provide a sufficient level of control for chance agreement, and states that fewer than five would be statistically unjustifiable. At the time that we were validating the content of our care pathways, no maximum number had been established. Therefore, the group contacted twelve experts, including continence nurse specialists, researchers and physiotherapists. Of course, there could be bias in the sample if the experts were selected from colleagues of the care pathways development group. To avoid this skew in the sample, the experts selected were not personally known to the development group, to ensure that the experts were independent and had no immediate, invested interest in the project.

The individuals were initially approached to see whether they wanted to be involved. Once they had agreed to take part, they were sent a pack containing both the pathways they were to validate and validation sheets. The experts were asked to bring to the task their beliefs and values as to whether the pathways were good practice that would benefit the patients. They were asked to validate the following documents:

■ continence assessment
■ symptom profile
■ care pathway for stress incontinence
■ care pathway for urge incontinence
■ care pathway for overflow continence

The validation process entailed subjecting the pathways to content validity testing, a method that is rarely used in the development of pathways (Anders *et al.*, 1997). The content validity method devised by Lynn (1986) involved two stages for the experts, each stage being set out on different validation sheets. The first stage required consideration of each statement within the pathway and the ranking of its validity according to the relevance of the approach to clinical care and good practice. The ranking was from 1 to 4, where 1 = not relevant, 2 = unable to assess relevance without item revision, or item is in need of such revision it would no longer be relevant, 3 = relevant with minor alteration and 4 = very relevant and succinct. The experts were asked to comment when they deemed a statement to be invalid (that is where it was rated 1 or 2).

The second stage of the content validity method involved the consideration of each pathway as a whole and an assessment of its validity. There was a validation sheet with each of the pathways listed, along with the assessment and symptom profile. Once again, validity was to be ranked according to the relevance of the approach to clinical care and to good practice. The ranking from 1 to 4 was the same as the statements. Written comments were also requested when a pathway was considered to be invalid (that where it was rated 1 or 2).

The experts' response rate was 100%. Those approached were keen to be involved in what many referred to as an 'exciting and innovative project'. The analysis consisted of the validation of each item within each pathway and the validation of each pathway as a whole. To validate the results experts had to respond with scores of 3 or 4 to indicate that the item/whole pathway was relevant to that issue of care. The exact number of experts that had to respond positively to an item/whole pathway for it to be validated was calculated using the Content Validity Index (Lynn, 1986).

The validation process was intended to generate quantitative data, although, because the pathways were validated, of particular interest were the written comments that the experts had made. They had not limited themselves to commenting only where items were not validated but had written notes where they felt appropriate. These notes consisted of positive comments and constructive criticism. The development group spent some time going through these comments. The comments were used to inform the development of the pathways. Specific changes made included:

1. The pathway for stress incontinence required the completion of a symptom profile and continence assessment again on a second visit. This was unnecessary, as all that was needed was a bothersome rating. The simple comment that had triggered this change was 'Why?'

2. It was not made clear at what point to refer to the continence nurse specialist in the overflow pathway.
3. It was unclear at which points and for what aspect of care the assessing nurse was required to sign. This was clarified in all of the pathways.

All these seemingly small points, when assimilated, led to a re-design of the pathway, which resulted in lessening the amount of paperwork generated by the administering of the care pathways.

One issue that was less easy to resolve, at least immediately, involved the comments that were made by some of the experts to the time span of four to six weeks allowed between visits on the pathways for urge and stress incontinence. The experts were divided as to whether the visits should be more or less frequent. Their comments were grounded in the fact that they believed that for treatment to be effective patients should be visited more frequently; however, in reality, time and resource constraints do not permit more frequent visits.

Therefore, the period has remained the same, as the pathways development group has decided to see what is written in the box beside this item when the pathways are used in practice. Any period between visits that varies from four to six weeks should be recorded and if in, say, 50% of cases there is a variation then the item on the pathway will need to be altered. This is an example of the variance tracking that was intended as an integral part of the project and is illustrative of the pathways as a dynamic form. It is also a demonstration of how pathways can be adapted to local resources and needs.

Focus groups

The aim of these groups was to collect the views of users of continence services to help improve the quality of these services through the introduction of care pathways. There are issues to be aware of in undertaking focus groups. It may be that one person dominates the discussion, which will have the effect of others not being able to contribute as much as they could, and it is difficult or impossible to follow up the views of individual group members (Robson, 1993). In this instance, however, there were two main reasons for using such groups. First, working in groups is a good way of generating ideas. Second, incontinence is not necessarily an easy subject for people to talk about but focus group work can boost the confidence of participants once they realise they share common experiences.

The main aim of the focus group was to collect the views of participants on the paperwork to be used with care pathways and to generate ideas as to how it could be used to maximum effect. A secondary aim was to treat the focus group as an opportunity to get ideas for improving the continence service. The participants' views produced extremely useful material on the existing service, and on possible improvements to it, although this information adds little to the current discussion.

On the day of the focus group the eighteen participants were asked to work in small groups. On each task they were asked for their written comments first and then to share these comments with their groups. Groups are a good means of giving people with similar symptoms the confidence to share their experiences and learning that they are not alone. Each group had a facilitator, who was there to take them through the tasks, note comments on a flip chart and to facilitate discussion.

Patients had not before been asked quality-of-life questions, but following its research, the group had come up with two questions: *How much does your bladder problem bother you?* and *What is your expectation of the treatment?* Participants were asked to respond to and then discuss these questions.

They were then required to complete and comment on the symptom profile and urinary monitoring journal, and finally to read and comment on the patient information sheets.

Participants were asked to complete evaluation sheets, giving their ratings on certain features of the day. The comments made verbally about the day were confirmed in the evaluation sheets: 94% of the respondents thought the sessions either very good or excellent and all the respondents that events like this were useful. They found the event reassuring, as did the professionals and more particularly the continence care pathways development group, which had been a little apprehensive about asking users for their views for fear of what issues might be raised.

The question on the pathways that users were asked to comment on – *How much does your bladder problem bother you?* – was found to work well and patients were able to respond. However, the second question – *What is your expectation of the treatment?* – meant

Box 7.1 Focus group's views about continence services

- Lack of understanding of what the continence service is and what it has to offer (only one participant had heard of the service).
- The NHS is viewed as providing products and pads, not advice or treatment.
- In the use of care pathways it may be important to make it clear that the aims are to reduce symptoms wherever possible.
- Participants expected to receive advice on the best ways of coping rather than any suggestion of a cure.

little to them and they were unable to answer. After discussion, it was agreed that the first question should be rated (not at all, a little, moderately, a lot) supplemented by *What is the effect on your life of your continence problems?*, which would elicit better-quality information and could also be more readily understood. Box 7.1 lists some of the statements that the ensuing discussion about treatment included.

Respondents were asked to complete the symptom profile and then asked for their verbal comments. There were no major problems for individuals in completing the paperwork, only suggestions to make completion easier. At the top of the profile it was suggested it specify to read through all possible symptoms on the profile before ticking those most relevant to them, as some statements were quite similar. Other possible changes included leaving space for the patient/nurse to comment and to indicate that the colour coding is not important or for official use only.

The three groups were asked to complete different parts of the urinary journal. In sharing their views many points emerged from the discussions. Box 7.2 displays these suggestions made by the focus group for service improvements.

All changes as detailed in Box 7.2 have been incorporated into the care pathways.

How can user involvement be undertaken locally?

The *Improvement leaders' guide* entitled *Involving Patients and Carers* 'sets out the means of involving patients in health services'

Box 7.2 Focus group's suggestions for service improvements

- Clear and full explanation of the benefits prior to completion and thorough explanation of how the information informs the care after completion.
- Advice on how such information is used to treat incontinence.
- The journal to be targeted only at those who benefit the most, not at everyone.
- Ensure clarity of questions: difficulty in understanding leads to lack of compliance.
- Always offer feedback to those who fill out the journals, even if the patterns fall within normal ranges.
- Apparent lack of appreciation for work undertaken by patients will result in poor compliance with other health providers in the future.

(NHS Institute for Innovation and Improvement, 2005a). This involvement is seen as improving the patient journey through the health service and beyond, that is from feeling that something is wrong and going to the doctor, routine screening and staying well to maintaining quality of life. Patient involvement is also referred to in the context of process mapping, which is to do with service redesign and the use of models of good practice (as detailed in Chapter 3).

The following techniques may be used in the involvement of users (NHS Institute for Innovation and Improvement, 2005a).

Focus groups

In the development of the pathways we used this method to involve users. An interesting way that focus groups can be used is as what the *Leaders guide* terms 'patient as teacher'. The first stage of this process is to facilitate a focus group of patients, much like the one described above, within which users are asked questions about their illness and for suggestions as to how the service may be improved. The second stage comprises some of those who have taken part in the focus group volunteering to represent the entire focus group in meetings with doctors and nurses from the relevant services, and to use these meetings as opportunities to teach health care professionals good practice from the point of view of the patient by sharing with them suggestions for the improvement of the services that those professionals provide. The different parties involved would then work on devising and implementing a future plan of action to improve service outcomes for patients.

This technique would be useful for users of continence services where their condition is chronic and they have contact with the service over a long period of time.

Patient shadowing

Another patient, member of staff or volunteer follows a patient around as they present themselves to the health services to help understand and feedback how a service is performing and how it may improve. This method could be used in conjunction with other methods, such as interviews with staff, to give a balanced view of health care.

Patient shadowing would be best used where there is a process mapping exercise taking place and where it would give a full description of the patient journey. The findings could be used in staff training and to audit service performance.

Patient diaries

Patients may be asked to record events, timings and action relating to the service they receive as well as their feelings relating to the experience. They may be unstructured or require the participants to respond to specific questions. This is a broader recording than the urinary journal, which asks for patients to record their urinary symptoms.

Diaries are useful for collecting detailed information on the patient's perspective. They appear attractive because they potentially generate substantial amounts of data with relatively little input from the researcher. There are drawbacks, however. For example, there is the risk of misreporting, perhaps to please the researcher. Owing to such shortcomings, diaries are often used in conjunction with other methods. Diary-keeping was one data-collection technique used by Godfrey and Hogg (2007) in their study for Help the Aged concerning the impact of incontinence on the health and well-being of older patients. Twenty people with incontinence kept a diary for three days. Interviews were undertaken and the authors used the results from the diary analysis with data from the interviews to report that incontinence does have an impact on social involvement.

Discovery interviews

Interviews are undertaken with users and carers, usually in their own homes, to ascertain the patient's experience, and the interview is structured so as to get from the patient their story of the impact on their lives of their illness.

Because patients are involved, interviews, as well as all other techniques for getting the user's perspective, will require getting ethical approval. There are local ethics committees across the United Kingdom that would need to be approached for such information-gathering to take place. This approval will require obtaining the patient's consent and guaranteeing anonymity and confidentiality. Interviews can give a detailed account of a patient's experience of an illness and/or service and are particularly useful for generating rich descriptions (that is quotes) that can be used to subsequently represent users' accounts when presenting the findings of any investigation.

Critical friends groups

The formation of these groups starts with an audit of service provision administered to staff or users. A questionnaire is given to individuals who use the service, and they are asked to assess how well the service is performing. When the data are gathered, a few users are asked to meet with staff – a critical friends group – to discuss the findings and help identify future priorities for the service and likely solutions to any identified problems.

Critical friends groups work best when there is a good supportive relationship between staff delivering the service and users receiving it.

Which technique is used for involving patients will depend on what input from patients is required, but any or all of them will enable the reader to carry out their own audits and enable them to involve users in the process mapping and/or local adaptation of care pathways.

Key summary points

- Development of care pathways lends itself to patient/user involvement.
- Quality services respond better to the needs of patients.
- Patients can be involved through the Expert Patients Programme.
- There are different styles and types of user involvement.
- Pathway content should be validated.
- Patient involvement improves the patient journey through care.

Chapter 8

Resources

This chapter identifies where further information can be obtained. For both staff and patients there is an enormous amount of help and information available. This is largely because of increased access to the Internet, but the authors caution against the use of material which may be neither valid nor reliable and emphasise that educational material should not be used unless an evidence base can be provided for it.

There are organisations that have been formed to promote continence. Patients have formed patient support groups. Books, leaflets and videos for professionals, patients and carers have been produced. Commercial companies also offer educational materials and even provide telephone helplines.

It is impossible to provide a fully comprehensive guide here, but we have included a selection of sources of help, information, support and advice.

The first section includes organisations offering support to patients, carers and professionals. It includes organisations that provide information and advice about equipment. The second section includes details of companies that provide educational material. The third section covers resources on the Internet that are intended to help with the development of pathways and answer questions about how to involve patients. All websites were accessed in August 2008. Some of the websites refer to *integrated pathways*, which, although not the focus of this book, have been included here because some of the issues and discussion points are the same.

Organisations offering support to patients, carers and professionals

Digestive Disorders Foundation (Core)
St Andrews Place
London NW1 4LB

Telephone: 020 7486 0341
Website: http://www.corecharity.org.uk/

Core is the working name of the Digestive Disorders Foundation. The foundation is a charity which provides information and leaflets to help sufferers control their symptoms.

IBS Network
The Gut Trust
Unit 5
53 Mowbray Street
Sheffield S3 8EN

Telephone/helpline: 0114 272 3253
Website: http://www.ibsnetwork-org.uk

The IBS Network is a registered charity. It is a self-help organisation. Its website offers advice and information in a friendly and under-standable manner about irritable bowel syndrome. It has self-help groups nationwide.

Association for Continence Advice
C/o Fitwise Management Ltd
Drumcross Hall
Bathgate
West Lothian EH48 4JT

Telephone: 01506 811077
Website: http://www.aca.uk.com
Email: aca@fitwise.co.uk

The ACA is a multidisciplinary professional body open to all health and allied care professionals and to those who have a concern for the promotion of continence and the better management of incontinence.

ERIC (Education and Resources for Improving Childhood Continence)
34 Old School House
Britannia Road
Kingswood
Bristol BS15 8DB

Telephone: 0117 960 3060
Helpline: 0845 370 8008
Website: http://www.eric.org.uk

ERIC is a national children's health charity dealing with bedwetting, daytime wetting, constipation and soiling in children and young people. Eric provides information, support and resources to families and health professionals.

Bladder and Bowel Foundation (formerly Incontact and the Continence Foundation)
SATRA Innovation Park
Rockingham Road
Kettering
Northamptonshire NN16 9JH

Telephone: 01536 533255
Website: http://www.bladderandbowelfoundation.org
Nurse helpline: 0845 345 0165
Counsellor helpline: 0870 770 3246

The Bladder and Bowel Foundation is the United Kingdom's leading charity dedicated to supporting people living with bladder and bowel disorders. It provides information, advice and support for all types of bladder- and bowel-related problems for patients, their families and friends. For health care professionals and carers it provides information and support systems to help improve patient care. It has a dedicated specialist nurse helpline, providing clinical support for both patients and carers, and a counsellor helpline, providing advice and a sympathetic ear.

The International Continence Society (UK)
19 Portland Square
Bristol BS2 8SI

Telephone: 01179 444881
Website: http://www.icsoffice.org
Email: info@icsoffice.co.uk

The ICS is a multidisciplinary international society that holds an international research conference annually. It is a registered charity.

Continence Care Forum (for nurses)
20 Cavendish Square
London WI9 0RN

Telephone: 020 7409 3333
Website: http://www.rcn.org.uk

This is a specialist interest group within the Royal College of Nursing for nurses with an interest in continence. It supports continence nurse specialists.

The Association of Chartered Physiotherapists in Women's Health (ACPWH)
C/o Fitwise Management Ltd
Drumcross Hall
Bathgate
West Lothian EH48 4JT

Telephone: 01506 811077
Website: http://www.acpwh.org.uk

The ACPWH is a specialist interest group for physiotherapists.

Spinal Injuries Association
SIA House
2 Trueman Place
Oldbrook
Milton Keynes
Buckinghamshire MK6 2HH

Telephone: 0845 678 6633
Advice line: 0800 980 0501
Website: http://www.spinal.co.uk

The SIA offers support to people with spinal cord injuries.

The Princess Royal Trust for Carers

The Princess Royal Trust for Carers
Unit 14
Bourne Court
Southend Road
Woodford Green
Essex IG8 8HD

Telephone: 0844 800 4361
Website: http://www.carers.org/
Email: info@carers.org

The Princess Royal Trust for Carers provides comprehensive carer support throughout the United Kingdom via a network of centres.

Multiple Sclerosis Society

MS National Centre
372 Edgware Road
London NW2 6ND

Telephone: 020 8438 0700
Website: http://www.mssociety.org.uk

The Multiple Sclerosis Society is a registered charity that produces, for sufferers of multiple sclerosis, leaflets which give guidance on managing bladder and bowel problems.

The Cystitis and Overactive Bladder Foundation

76 High Street
Stony Stratford
Buckinghamshire MK11 1AH

Telephone: 01908 569169
Website: http://www.cobfoundation.org
Email: info@cobfoundation.org

The Cystitis and Overactive Bladder Foundation is a charity that provides information and support to sufferers of bladder problems, including interstitial cystitis, bacterial cystitis and overactive bladder.

Organisations that provide information and advice about equipment

Promocon
Redbank House
4 St Chads Street
Cheetham
Manchester M8 8QA

Telephone: 08707 601580
Telephone helpline: 0161 834 2001
Website: http://www.promocon.co.uk
Email: promocon@disabledliving.co.uk

Promocon is an information centre in Manchester with an exhibition of continence products. It gives independent advice and product information to both patients and professionals. It comes under the umbrella of Disabled Living and is moving in June 2009.

Assist UK
Redbank House
4 St Chads Street
Cheetham
Manchester M8 8QA

Telephone: 0870 770 2866
Website: http://assist-uk.org/
Email: general.info@assist-uk.org

Assist UK leads a UK-wide network of locally situated Disabled Living Centres. Each centre provides a permanent exhibition of products and equipment. People can try the equipment and get professional advice.

Royal Association for Disability and Rehabilitation (RADAR)
12 City Forum
250 City Road
London EC1V 8AF

Telephone: 020 7250 3222
Minicom: 020 7250 4119
Website: http://radar.org.uk
Email: radar@radar.org.uk

RADAR is a registered charity and a national network of disabled people and disability organisations. It offers information about a national key scheme for disabled toilets and accommodation that caters for people who suffer from a disability and a continence problem.

Remap
D9 Chaucer Business Park
Kemsing
Sevenoaks
Kent TN15 6YU

Telephone: 0845 1300 456
Website: http://www.remap.org.uk/

Remap custom makes equipment for people with disabilities.

Companies providing educational material

Norgine Limited
Chaplin House
Widewater Place
Moorhall Road
Harefield
Uxbridge
Middlesex UB9 6NS

Telephone: 01895 826 600
Email: mss@norgine.com

Norgine supplies the following helpful publications:

- *Graphic diagram: Correct position for opening your bowels:* This simple chart describes the correct position for defecation. It can be used as a poster or handout.
- *Bristol Stool Form Scale:* This was produced to enable the correct titration of medication. It is also an evidence-based tool for aiding the completion of bowel diaries by patients.
- *The procedure for the digital removal of faeces:* This booklet sets out the procedure for the digital removal of faeces, and was produced in partnership with the Association for Continence Advice, the Royal College of Nursing and the Spinal Injuries Association. It includes information on digital stimulation.

- *Risk assessment tool for constipation:* This identifies which patients may be at risk of constipation, using the following indicators: medical condition, medication, environment, mobility, nutrition and fluid intake.
- *Impact paediatric bowel care pathway:* This details a care pathway for children with bowel problems.
- *Practical procedures: Bowel care (CD-ROM):* This deals with the assessment of constipation, the assessment of functional constipation in children, obtaining a stool sample, administering an enema, administering a suppository, and has a practical guide to digital rectal examination and Bristol Stool Form Scales (adult and child).

Astra Tech Ltd
Brunel Way
Stonehouse
Gloucestershire GL10 2HH

Telephone: 0800 652 3350
Website: http://www.lofric.co.uk

Astra Tech produces the following helpful publications:
Professional:

- *ISC Nurses Guide*

Professional and user:

- *Patient Checklist* (works with health care professionals)
- *Living with LoFric guides*
- *Spinal cord injury guides*
- *Standard LoFric user leaflet*
- *Bladder Health in Neurological Conditions*

Astellas Pharma Limited
Lovett House
Lovett Road
Staines TW18 3AZ

Telephone: 01784 419615
Website (for patient use only): http://astellas-vip.co.uk/

Information for patients:

- *Helpful Hints Leaflet:* Information on bladder retraining, fluid intake and pelvic floor exercises
- *Vesicare information programme:* As above, plus in DVD form, includes reminders and **should only be viewed by patients who have been prescribed solifenacin.**

SCA Personal Care
Southfields Road
Dunstable
Bedfordshire LU6 3EJ

Telephone (TENA advice line for consumers): 0845 30 80 80 30
Website: http://www.tenanet.co.uk

SCA Personal Care produces the *Continence Promotion Resource Pack.* This collection of useful, evidence-based educational material, including some useful references, and up-to-date research on incontinence management is available to all customers to support their continence promotion work. The TENA Net extranet site is a resource containing news on the latest developments relating to incontinence and can be used to download literature and order samples, and has a message board where customers can exchange best practice and find answers from their peers.

Educational literature

Leaflets and booklets are available from SCA Personal Care (listed above) on a wide range of subjects to support health care professionals and provide relevant information to patients. Below is a list of those available:

- Pelvic floor exercises for men
- Pelvic floor exercises for women
- A healthy bowel
- A healthy bladder
- Looking after your skin
- Product fitting guides
- Product fitting DVD
- Corewellness DVD
- COSSH sheets for all our skincare products

Website resources on care pathways and patient involvement

National Library for Health
Website: http://www.library.nhs.uk/pathways/AboutUs.aspx

On this website, use the search function to enter 'pathways' to search evidence-based reviews, guidance, specialist libraries, books, journals and health care databases. One of the specialist libraries is referred to below (that is the Protocols and Care Pathways Library).

On the same site, there is material on patient and public involvement (http://www.library.nhs.uk/ppi/). This website provides up-to-date policy and outlines what is going on nationally.

The Protocols and Care Pathways Library
Website: http://www.library.nhs.uk/Pathways/ViewResource.aspx?resID=259091&tabID=290&catID=12584

The Protocols and Care Pathways Library aims to provide information relating to the development and implementation of care pathways and protocols. The site has an extensive database of examples, which is maintained by the University of Birmingham. This website gives guidance on developing care pathways.

The King's Fund
Website: http://www.kingsfund.org.uk/information_and_library_service/reading_lists/index.html

This website has a great many reading lists, made up of books, reports, articles and Web resources on a wide range of topics, including patient decision-making, patient choice, Patient Advice & Liaison Services (PALS) and care pathways.

European Pathway Association
Website: http://www.e-p-a.org/index2.html

The European Pathway Association is an international network of researchers, managers and clinicians who want to share knowledge on the health care management concept of clinical/care pathways, pathways education, running conferences undertaking research and disseminating information.

e-Health Nurses Network

Website: http://www.ehealthnurses.org.uk

The aim of this network is 'to facilitate professional development through the exploration of e-health and its impact on patient care within a new, collaborative environment'. There is discussion specifically on e-pathways and their implications for nurses.

18 Weeks

Website: http://www.18weeks.nhs.uk/Content.aspx?path=/

The 18-week 'referral to treatment' pathway is about improving patients' experience of the NHS by ensuring all patients receive high-quality, elective care without any unnecessary delay. The organisation's name applies to pathways that do or may involve consultant-led care, setting a maximum time of 18 weeks from the point of initial referral to the start of any treatment necessary for all patients where it is clinically appropriate and where patients want it.

NHS Institute for Innovation and Improvement

Website: http://www.institute.nhs.uk/

The NHS Institute for Innovation and Improvement supports the NHS to transform health care for patients and the public by rapidly developing and spreading new ways of working, new technology and world-class leadership. It produces useful management guides, like those referred to previously in this book (for example NHS Institute for Innovation and Improvement, 2005a: *Improvement leaders' guide: Involving patients and carers*). It is possible to search 'pathways' on the website for further information.

The Expert Patients Programme

Website: http://www.expertpatients.nhs.uk

The Expert Patients Programme is a lay-led self-management programme that has been specifically developed for people living with long-term conditions. The aim of the programme is to support people to increase their confidence, improve their quality of life and better manage their condition. (From Department of Health website, http://www.dh.gov.uk/en/Aboutus/ MinistersandDepartmentLeaders/ChiefMedicalOfficer/ProgressOnPolicy/ ProgressBrowsableDocument/DH_4102757)

This programme is detailed in Chapter 7 on patient and other expert involvement.

Venture Training & Consulting
Website: http://www.venturetc.com

This is an organisation dedicated to the development and support of integrated care pathways (ICPs) and has developed the first electronic ICP application (Nimbus Pathway). The software supports the planning, design, writing, implementation, variance tracking, analysis and reporting of ICPs as part of the electronic patient record (EPR).

Appendix 1

Information sheets for patients

The following information sheets are replicated here as examples of the types of sheets which may be given to patients.

They are:

1. Information sheet for women (pelvic floor/urgency)
2. Information sheet for men (pelvic floor/urgency)
3. Continence in the confused older person: information for carers
4. Caffeine: advice and alternatives
5. Looking after your bowels
6. Fibre content of everyday foods

They are suggested only as examples. Many companies who manufacture products and medication to help with incontinence produce such information sheets for patients and will provide these on request, free of charge.

Information sheet 1

Information sheet for women

Leakage when you cough, sneeze, run, jump or laugh may be called *stress incontinence*. It can be caused or aggravated by childbirth, being overweight, constipated or by chronic coughing. It is due to a weakness of the pelvic floor muscles. It is important that you do not reduce your fluid intake to try to control the leakage, as this may actually make your problem worse, and cause constipation.

Urgency is the symptom of having to hurry to pass urine. Whatever the cause, there are certain rules to follow to help control your symptoms.

- Do not reduce your fluid intake. Far from helping, this may make your problem much worse, and can cause constipation.
- Try to avoid drinks containing caffeine, which is found in tea, coffee, chocolate and cola.
- Fizzy drinks may exacerbate symptoms.
- Alcohol can also increase urgency.
- Avoid passing urine 'just in case'.
- Try to increase the amount of time between visits to the toilet.
- Do not try to hold on at night: it will only keep you awake. Practising holding on in the daytime will gradually help night-time problems.
- If you have been given water tablets, you must take them no matter how often they make you want to go. Discuss this problem with your nurse or doctor.
- If you are overweight, try to lose a few pounds; this will relieve stress on the pelvic floor.
- Be careful with your diet: too much or too little fibre is not good for you. Try changing your diet to see what works best for you.

Physiotherapists, doctors and nurses know that pelvic floor exercises can help you to improve your bladder control. When done correctly, pelvic floor exercises can build up and strengthen the muscles to help you to hold urine.

Pelvic floor exercises for women

The pelvic floor

Layers of muscle stretch like a hammock from the pubic bone, at the front, to the bottom of the backbone, at the back. These firm, supportive muscles are called *the pelvic floor*. They help to hold the bladder, womb and bowel in place, and to close the bladder outlet and back passage. The pelvic floor muscles are linked by nerve pathways with the lower abdominal muscles (*transversus abdominus*) and the interior back muscles (*multifidus*). This means that these three muscle groups work together and support each other. They work together to maintain good posture of the pelvis, which is very important as the pelvic floor muscles rely on this to maintain their tone.

How the pelvic floor works

The muscles of the pelvic floor are kept firm and slightly tense to stop leakage of urine from the bladder or faeces from the bowel. This is where the posture of the pelvis is important. If the lower abdominal muscles are relaxed, it will be difficult for the pelvic floor to be firm, and make it slightly tense. When you pass water or have a bowel motion, the pelvic floor muscles relax. Afterwards, they tighten again to restore control. When you cough, sneeze or laugh, it triggers a reflex which automatically tightens the pelvic floor strongly.

Pelvic floor muscles can become weak and sag because of childbirth, lack of exercise and poor posture, the change of life or just from getting older. Weak muscles give you less control, and you may leak urine, especially with exercise or when you cough, sneeze or laugh.

How pelvic floor exercises can help

Pelvic floor exercises can strengthen these muscles so that they can again give support. Once you understand how to use the pelvic floor, you will be able to support the automatic reflex when you cough, sneeze or laugh.

Pelvic floor exercises can strengthen these muscles so that they once again give support. This will improve your bladder control and improve or stop leakage of urine. Like any other muscles in the body, the more you use and exercise them, the stronger the pelvic floor will be.

How to do your pelvic floor exercises

It is important that your pelvis be held in the right position to help the pelvic floor to work most efficiently with its co-workers. These are the *transversus abdominus* and the *multifidus*.

Centred pelvic posture

Stand normally in front of a mirror if possible. Think about standing as tall as you can, imagine a balloon floating above your head, which is pulling you up with it. As you grow taller tuck your bottom in and pull your pubic bone up at the front. Your tummy should look flatter in the mirror but you should be able to breathe normally. This good posture helps to maintain the postural tension in the pelvic floor muscles and will help to give your muscles a continuous workout.

In addition to improving postural tension you will need to do extra exercises for the pelvic floor to improve your control and strength.

THE LIFT

- Whilst assuming good posture (either sitting or standing), tighten the muscle around the anus (back passage). Imagine you are trying to stop wind from escaping!
- Now try the same exercise with the front part of the muscle. This part of the muscle is just behind the pubic bone and lifts the entrance to the vagina. This exercise is more difficult and takes time to master.
- Once you have identified the two groups of muscles and can confidently tighten them together, you are ready to start exercising them. You should try to tighten as hard as you can for as long as possible. This may initially be for only a few seconds. You can build this up to five to ten seconds. It is a good idea to link the lift with the activities you do. For instance, every time you pick up something in your right hand (if you are right-handed), tighten the pelvic floor. This makes the exercise more functional and natural. Research tells us that contracting the pelvic floor 100+ times daily will strengthen the pelvic floor. If you do the lift every time you pick up something in your hand, you will be doing the exercise many more times than 100+ daily! Remember: when you pick up, tighten up!

THE WINK

- Try to 'wink' the pelvic floor muscles in a one-second flick, then relax. Repeat this five to 10 times.
- Working the muscles in the lift and the wink – slowly and then fast – will strengthen and improve control of the pelvic floor.

So you are now working hard at these exercises and busy improving your posture, but there is one more thing for you to learn. It is a trick, where timing and strength is important and can help you control leakage when you cough, sneeze or laugh. It will help you to support your automatic reflex.

THE TRICK

When you need to cough, sneeze or laugh, tighten the pelvic floor muscles a couple of times, to wake them up, then tighten strongly just at the moment when you cough, sneeze or laugh. Then relax. Timing is important! That is why it is essential that you practise the lift and the wink, as doing these exercises will lead to better control and improved strength.

To practise the trick tighten the pelvic floor as described above, take a breath and 'huff' the air out of your lungs sharply or you can try a small cough. Remember to keep the pelvic floor tight. Remember to have good posture.

You may find pelvic floor exercises and improving your posture difficult at first, but you will need patience and perseverance to improve. All exercise needs to be repeated regularly in order to get a good result and the pelvic floor is no exception. You may notice an improvement within six to eight weeks if you perform the exercises as above. The exercises will become easier to perform as the pelvic floor becomes stronger and more controlled and it will soon become a habit to tighten whenever you pick anything up in your hand.

Remember: when you pick up, tighten up.

Information sheet 2

Information sheet for men

Urgency is the symptom of having to hurry to pass urine. Whatever the cause, there are certain rules to follow to help control your symptoms.

- Do not reduce your fluid intake. Far from helping, this may make your problem much worse, and can cause constipation.
- Try to avoid drinks containing caffeine, which is found in tea, coffee, chocolate and cola.

- Fizzy drinks may exacerbate symptoms.
- Alcohol can also increase urgency.
- Avoid passing urine 'just in case'.
- Try to increase the amount of time between visits to the toilet.
- Do not try to hold on at night: it will only keep you awake. Practising holding on in the daytime will gradually help night-time problems.
- If you have been given water tablets, you must take them no matter how often they make you want to go. Discuss this problem with your nurse or doctor.
- If you are overweight, try to lose a few pounds; this will relieve stress on the pelvic floor.
- Be careful with your diet: too much or too little fibre is not good for you. Try changing your diet to see what works best for you.

Physiotherapists, doctors and nurses know that pelvic floor exercises can help you to improve your bladder control. When done correctly, pelvic floor exercises can build up and strengthen the muscles to help you to hold urine.

Do not feel embarrassed by this problem: studies show that more men suffer with this than you would think.

Pelvic floor exercises for men

The pelvic floor

Layers of muscle stretch like a hammock from the pubic bone, at the front, to the bottom of the backbone, at the back. These firm, supportive muscles are called *the pelvic floor*. They help to hold the bladder and bowel in place, and to close the bladder outlet and back passage. The pelvic floor muscles are linked by nerve pathways with the lower abdominal muscles (*transversus abdominus*) and the interior back muscles (*multifidus*). This means that these three muscle groups work together and support each other. They work together to maintain good posture of the pelvis, which is very important as the pelvic floor muscles rely on this to maintain their tone.

How the pelvic floor works

The muscles of the pelvic floor are kept firm and slightly tense to stop leakage of urine from the bladder or faeces from the bowel.

This is where the posture of the pelvis is important. If the lower abdominal muscles are relaxed, it will be difficult for the pelvic floor to be firm, and make it slightly tense. When you pass water or have a bowel motion, the pelvic floor muscles relax. Afterwards, they tighten again to restore control. When you cough, sneeze or laugh, it triggers a reflex, which automatically tightens the pelvic floor strongly.

Pelvic floor muscles can become weak and sag because of childbirth, lack of exercise and poor posture, the change of life or just from getting older. Weak muscles give you less control, and you may leak urine, especially with exercise or when you cough, sneeze or laugh.

How pelvic floor exercises can help

Pelvic floor exercises can strengthen these muscles so that they can again give support. Once you understand how to use the pelvic floor, you will be able to support the automatic reflex when you cough, sneeze or laugh. This will improve your bladder control and improve or stop leakage of urine. Like any other muscle in the body, the more you use and exercise them, the stronger the pelvic floor will be.

How to do your pelvic floor exercises

It is important that your pelvis be held in the right position to help the pelvic floor to work most efficiently with its co-workers. These are the *transversus abdominus* and the *multifidus*.

Centred pelvic posture

Stand normally, in front of a mirror if possible. Think about standing as tall as you can, imagine a balloon floating above your head, which is pulling you up with it. As you grow taller tuck your bottom in and pull your pubic bone up at the front. Your tummy should look flatter in the mirror but you should be able to breathe normally. You may notice that your anus tightens; this is because the anus is part of the pelvic floor muscles. This good posture helps to maintain the postural tension in the pelvic floor muscles and will help to give your muscles a continuous workout.

In addition to improving postural tension you will need to do extra exercises for the pelvic floor to improve your control and strength.

THE LIFT

- Whilst assuming good posture (either sitting or standing), tighten the muscle around the anus (back passage). Imagine you are trying to stop wind from escaping!
- Now try the same exercise with the front part of the muscle. This part of the muscle is just behind the pubic bone and lifts the penis. This exercise is more difficult and takes time to master.
- Once you have identified the two groups of muscles and can confidently tighten them together, you are ready to start exercising them. You should try to tighten as hard as you can for as long as possible. This may initially be for only a few seconds. You can build this up to five to ten seconds. It is a good idea to link the lift with the activities you do. For instance, every time you pick up something in your right hand (if you are right-handed), tighten the pelvic floor. This makes the exercise more functional and natural. Research tells us that contracting the pelvic floor 100+ times daily will strengthen the pelvic floor. If you do the lift every time you pick up something in your hand, you will be doing the exercise many more times than 100+ daily! Remember: when you pick up, tighten up!

THE WINK

- Try to 'wink' the pelvic floor muscles in a one-second flick, then relax. Repeat this five to 10 times.
- Working the muscles in the lift and the wink – slowly and then fast – will strengthen and improve control of the pelvic floor.

So you are now working hard at these exercises and busy improving your posture, but there is one more thing for you to learn. It is a trick, where timing and strength is important and can help you control leakage when you cough, sneeze or laugh. It will help you to support your automatic reflex.

THE TRICK

When you need to cough, sneeze or laugh, tighten the pelvic floor muscles a couple of times, to wake them up, then tighten strongly just at the moment when you cough, sneeze or laugh. Then relax.

Timing is important! That is why it is essential that you practise the lift and the wink, as doing these exercises will lead to better control and improved strength.

To practise the trick tighten the pelvic floor as described above, take a breath and 'huff' the air out of your lungs sharply or you can try a small cough. Remember to keep the pelvic floor tight. Remember to have good posture.

You may find pelvic floor exercises and improving your posture difficult at first, but you will need patience and perseverance to improve. All exercise needs to be repeated regularly in order to get a good result and the pelvic floor is no exception. You may notice an improvement within six to eight weeks if you perform the exercises as above. The exercises will become easier to perform as the pelvic floor becomes stronger and more controlled and it will soon become a habit to tighten whenever you pick anything up in your hand.

Remember: when you pick up, tighten up.

Information sheet 3

Continence in the confused older person: information for carers

Being demented: a human being imprisoned in a damaged brain.

The way we stay continent is a very complex function that allows us to voluntarily postpone passing urine or having our bowels opened until we are at the appropriate place. This skill can be affected by a dementing illness. It may happen just occasionally or, as the illness progresses, more frequently.

It is very important to understand that it may be due to a treatable condition so the first thing to do is discuss it with a health care professional.

Treatable conditions

Treatable conditions may include:

- *Urinary tract infection (UTI):* someone may complain of pain or burning when passing water or may show an expression of pain if they have difficulty talking. You or the person may notice that their urine looks cloudy or smells. Sometimes an infection can be present without specific symptoms so it is always worthwhile asking your nurse or doctor to check that all is well.

- *Prostate gland trouble (in men):* your GP will be able to assess whether this is a problem and advise you about treatment and help in managing leakage.
- *The side effects of some medication:* unfortunately, some medications do affect how your bladder and bowel work. It is always advisable to discuss this with your doctor if this could be the case and he or she may be able to change them or alter the dose.

Please take advice before stopping or changing when you take any medicines.

- *Severe constipation* may cause urinary incontinence through pressure on the bladder or bowel leakage, where loose, smelly motion leaks round the hard stool blocking the bowel. It is important that you discuss this with a health care professional, who can advise you on how to improve this problem. It is very important to try to help this person keep their own continence skills for as long as possible.
- *Lack of recall:* sadly, when people become forgetful, they may gradually lose the memory of what to do in a toilet or even where the toilet is. Advice can be given to help you manage in these circumstances.

How you can help

- *Get to know the person's habits.* This may seem a strange and very personal thing to suggest but usually our bladder and bowel actions have some pattern to them, and so it may be worthwhile noting when the person is most likely to use the toilet. As their memory starts to play tricks on them, you can help by reminding them to go to the toilet at the times when you know they are most likely to go. Keep this as a regular routine.
- *Learn to read the signs.* It may be that the person finds it difficult to verbally let you know they need to use a toilet. If this is the case, you will need to become aware of other signs (such as fidgeting, wandering or pulling at clothing) to prompt you as to when to suggest they use the toilet.

- *Fluid intake.* Make sure they drink enough during the day to keep the bladder and bowels healthy. People can forget to drink, or be reluctant to. Their nurse or GP can advise you.
- *Stick to a routine.* When you think about it, using the toilet is a very complicated thing to do, involving as it does lots of different steps to be successful. Try to keep using the toilet to a few, regular, easy steps. Use the same language to ask or describe what is happening and keep to the same routine inside the toilet.
- *Decide the toilet routine, keep to it and tell others.* This is important so that when the person spends time apart from you the routine is the same and the skill is encouraged to remain.
- *Keep in contact with the health care professional who is helping you.* Discussing and monitoring changes as they occur can help prevent them from becoming larger problems.
- *Consider installing equipment.* There are many aids and adaptions that can make using the toilet easier. Talk to a health care professional, particularly an occupation therapist or physiotherapist, about these.
- *Get advice about clothing.* Consider adapting clothing so that the person can get quick access to themselves in the toilet (e.g. Velcro rather than zips or buttons). An occupational therapist can help you with this.
- *Help maintain a healthy diet.* Get advice about a diet that will keep the person's bowels healthy. Ask your nurse or doctor for help.
- *Get advice about special problems.* Aim to get help to manage any wetness and to keep the person dignified, comfortable and dry.
- *Don't you forget about you.* Take some time for yourself, and speak with friends and health care professionals about your worries, and use them as sounding boards or even just as someone to lean on from time to time.

Information sheet 4

Caffeine: advice and alternatives

Caffeine causes frequency of urination and an urgent need to void. Many patients suffering from these symptoms will find improvement if they eliminate caffeine from their diet. The purpose of this sheet is to give you information about where caffeine is found and what alternatives you can try.

What is caffeine?

Caffeine is a drug found in tea, coffee, cocoa, chocolate and cola. It is also used in a range of painkillers and cold remedies. Caffeine is a stimulant which acts directly on the heart and central nervous system. It can increase alertness but also causes insomnia. People who have a regular intake of caffeine will become addicted. However, even a relatively low caffeine intake will affect the bladder of a susceptible person.

Caffeine withdrawal

Users of caffeinated drinks and food types will often feel the effects of caffeine withdrawal. Symptoms can be in the form of headache, anxiety, difficulty in concentrating, drowsiness or muscular stiffness. The most common symptom is headache, which is reported by 50% of people who withdraw from caffeine use.

This sheet contains advice which will help you minimise the effects of cutting out caffeine.

Many people report success by cutting down caffeine at the rate of 50–100 mg per day. This is known as *caffeine fading*. The best way to proceed is to write down your caffeine intake for one week, then reduce your caffeine intake as above. Remember: you *must not* reduce your fluid intake but have substitutes readily available.

You can stop immediately. Withdrawal symptoms are more marked this way. Regular caffeine consumption reduces sensitivity to caffeine. When intake is reduced, the body becomes oversensitive to adenosine. As a response to this the blood pressure drops dramatically, leading to a headache. This usually lasts from one to five days and can be alleviated with painkillers, as long as you avoid those which include caffeine. This headache, which is well known amongst strong and heavy coffee drinkers, will also be alleviated by an intake of caffeine. In research abstinence from doses as low as 100 mg per day produced symptoms, but generally the higher the consumption, the more likely you are to have withdrawal symptoms.

Urinary symptoms will regress within a week or so. It will help you to keep a diary of your symptoms in order that you can compare before and after.

Caffeine content

The following tables show caffeine content for the average serving.

Coffee: milligrams per average serving

Type	Milligrams
Filter coffee	115–175
Brewed coffee	80–135
Instant coffee	65–100
Espresso coffee (single portion)	100
Brewed decaf. coffee	3–4
Instant decaf. coffee	2–3

Tea: milligrams per average serving

Type	Milligrams
Brewed, average	60
Instant	30
Green tea	25–60
Decaf.	2
Redbush, herbal and fruit	Nil
Cocoa	15
Drinking chocolate	5–15

Cold drinks: milligrams per can

Type	Milligrams
Red Bull	80
Coca Cola	34
Cherry, lemon vanilla coke	34
Diet Coke, diet lemon, lime, vanilla	46
Dr Pepper/diet Dr Pepper	41
Pepsi Cola	37
Diet Pepsi	36
Slimfast cappuccino flavour	40
Slimfast chocolate flavour	20
Mountain Dew	55
Chocolate milkshake	8

Food items: milligrams per average serving

Type	Milligrams
1 oz (28 g) Cadbury chocolate	15
1 oz (28 g) white chocolate	2–4
1 oz (28 g) plain chocolate	25
2 tbs chocolate sauce	5

Medications: average milligrams per dose

Type	Milligrams per dose
Anadin Extra (two tablets)	90
Lemsip Max	50
Solpadeine Headache	130
Beechams Flu Plus	50
Boots Cold and Flu Relief tablets	60
Hedex Extra	130
Syndol	60
Veganin	60
Alka Seltzer XS	80

Some interesting facts

- Herbal and fruit teas are caffeine-free.
- It is believed that caffeine works on the kidney in a similar way to water-retention tablets, and may have a direct effect on the relaxation of the bladder muscle.
- Australia has a limit of 145 mg of caffeine per litre of fluid.
- In parts of northern Thailand caffeine is illegal.
- Dark-roast coffee has more caffeine than light-roast by weight as the water loss is faster than the caffeine loss.
- Light-roast coffee has more caffeine than dark-roast by volume because the beans expand as they roast.
- Caffeine is present in tea leaves and coffee beans to the extent of about 4%. Tea also contains theobromine, as does chocolate, and the darker the chocolate, the higher the content. Theobromine is highly toxic to dogs and kills many each year.
- Physical dependence on caffeine can occur in as little as three days.
- 90 million cups of coffee are consumed in the United Kingdom every day.

- Guarana soda pop is very popular in Brazil. It contains 250 mg of caffeine.
- There is a significant association between drinking caffeinated coffee and decreasing bone mineral density. However, this can be countered by drinking one glass of milk each day to avoid osteoporosis.

Information sheet 5

Looking after your bowels

Did you know. . . ?

1. Drinking the correct amount of fluid for your body weight can help avoid constipation. The job of the last part of the gut is to absorb fluid back into the body; it will do this even if you are drinking very little. If you are not drinking enough, this makes the waste hard and so difficult to expel. Fluid helps the waste to remain slippery and therefore easier to pass.

   1.1 I need to drink.......cups/mugs of................per day.

2. *It is important to make sure that your diet has adequate fibre in it.* The best advice is to eat five portions of fruit and vegetables a day to maintain a healthy diet. Your nurse has a useful fibre-scoring sheet for you to see how much you are really eating.

   1.2 Fibre score: ....

   1.3 I need to consider this advice to improve my fibre: ....

3. Limber up! Regular exercise, within your limitations, can stimulate the bowel to work regularly.

4. It is important to be in a good position to have your bowels open so. . . *are you sitting comfortably?* This means being well supported and feeling safe, not slipping or sliding or having trouble getting on and off the toilet.

   1.4 Your nurse can help you access aids and adaptions to help.

5. Bowels benefit from routine. *Allow yourself time and privacy to empty your bowels.* This can be difficult if you require help and assistance in the toilet, but discuss this with your nurse; they may have some ideas to help.

6. *When you feel the need to empty your bowel – respond!* If you keep ignoring the bowel, you can make yourself constipated.
7. *Some* medicines you take may upset your bowel habit. *Do not stop medication, but* ask your nurse, doctor or pharmacist if you suspect this, for advice.

Fibre scoring sheet

Rate your diet for fibre

Pick the foods you eat at home and find your score, using the following table.

Score	1	2	3	Write your score here
Bread	White	Brown	Wholemeal/ granary	
Breakfast cereal (3 times per week or more)	Rarely or never eat or eat sugar-coated cereal (e.g. Frosties)	Corn Flakes Rice Crispies Cheerios Special K	Bran Flakes Weetabix Shredded Wheat Muesli Shreddies	
Potatoes, pasta and rice	Rarely or never eat	Eat potatoes, white rice or pasta most days	Eat potatoes in jackets, brown rice or pasta most days	
Pulses, beans and nuts	Rarely or never eat	Once a week or less	Three times a week or more	
Vegetables (all kinds other than pulses, potatoes and beans)	Less than once a week	1–3 times per week	Daily	
Fruit (all kinds)	Less than once a week	1–3 times per week	Daily	
Your total score				

Use the following score as a guide for future fibre intake:
0–12 = increase your fibre intake; 13–17 = good; 18 = excellent.

Information sheet 6

Fibre content of everyday foods

Fibre content of bread and flour

Type	Serving size (grams)	Fibre content (grams)
Wholemeal bread	25	1.5
Brown bread	25	0.9
Hovis bread	25	0.8
White bread	25	0.4
Wholemeal flour	25	2.3
Brown flour	25	1.6
White flour	25	0.8

Fibre content of breakfast cereals

Type	Serving size (grams)	Fibre content (grams)
All Bran	40	9.6
Bran Buds	40	8.8
Bran Flakes	30	3.9
Sultana Bran	30	3.0
Fruit 'n' Fibre	30	2.1
Country Store	30	1.8
Raisin Splitz	30	2.7
Cornflakes	30	0.3
Muesli	40	2.6
Oatmeal (raw)	25	0.8

Fibre content of nuts

Type	Serving size (grams)	Fibre content (grams)
Almonds	25	1.9
Brazils	25	1.1
Chestnuts	25	1.1
Hazelnuts	25	1.6
Coconut	25	1.8
Peanuts	25	1.6
Peanut butter	25	1.4
Walnuts	25	0.9

Fibre content of biscuits and pastry

Type	Serving size (grams)	Fibre content (grams)
Crispbread (rye)	25	2.9
Digestive	12	0.3
Gingernuts	12	0.2
Oatcakes	25	1.5
Shortbread	25	0.5
Short pastry	50	1.1

Fibre content of vegetables

Type	Serving size (grams)	Fibre content (grams)
Carrots	75	1.9
Beetroot	75	1.9
Swedes	75	2.6
Potatoes (jacket)	100	1.4
Potatoes (new)	100	1.1
Potatoes (peeled and boiled)	100	1.2
Spinach	100	1.6
Broccoli tops	100	3.0
Spring greens	100	3.6
Sprouts	100	4.8
Cabbage (cooked)	90	1.6
Cabbage (raw)	90	2.2
Cauliflower	90	1.4
Celery (raw)	30	0.3
Leeks	80	1.4
Lettuce	30	0.3
Peas (frozen)	65	3.3
Peas (canned)	85	4.1
Peas (fresh)	65	2.9
Broad beans	120	7.8
Butter beans	60	2.8
Baked beans	135	5.0
Runner beans	90	1.7
French beans	90	3.7
Lentils (split)	120	2.3
Corn on the cob	125	1.6
Sweetcorn (can)	60	0.8
Tomatoes (raw)	85	0.9
Onions	60	1.0

Fibre content of raw and cooked fruit

Type	Serving size (grams)	Fibre content (grams)
Eating apples	100	1.8
Avocado pear	75	2.6
Banana	100	1.1
Blackberries	100	3.1
Cherries	100	0.9
Dates – dried	15	0.5
Figs – dried	20	1.5
Black grapes	100	0.7
Grapefruit	80	1.0
Melon	150	1.5
Orange	160	2.7
Peach	110	1.7
Pear	170	3.7
Raisins	24	0.5
Raspberries	60	1.5
Strawberries	100	1.1
Sultanas	24	0.5
Pineapple	80	1.0
Blackcurrants[a]	140	3.9
Gooseberries[a]	140	2.7
Plums[a]	140	1.7
Prunes[a]	24	0.6
Rhubarb[a]	140	1.7

[a] Cooked with sugar

Appendix 2

Information sheets for staff using pathways

The following information sheets for staff are presented as examples.

1. What is a care pathway? Information for new users
2. Medications affecting urinary continence status
3. Medications which may be associated with constipation
4. Abdominal massage
5. Laxatives
6. Autonomic dysreflexia
7. Neurogenic bowel management
8. Neurogenic bowel responses
9. Normal bowel habits
10. Bowel diary
11. Symptoms and causes of obstruction
12. Constipation: signs and symptoms

Information sheet 1

What is a care pathway? Information for new users

A care pathway (CP) is a tool to help provide the best possible evidence-based care. These CPs are based upon an extensive literature review of the most up-to-date evidence of best continence care. They set out the actions and stages of care in document form that staff can use as their clinical record of care. The CP is designed as a guide for professionals to follow, with prompts and triggers when referrals to other agencies should be sought and reminders of what actions need to be taken. However, your individual patient is unique and the CP should not be followed blindly. Professional judgement and consideration of the patient's individual needs must be taken into account. If the standard statement is not appropriate, then you can vary from the care prescribed by completing the variance tracking section of the document.

It cannot be emphasised how important it is to complete the variance from care: the analysis of this can lead to clear identification of resource issues, review of care and changes in the CP as a whole.

Regular variance tracking will take place and feedback will be given. This is what makes the CP dynamic and will always be up to date with local issues, research and good clinical practice.

This assessment must be carried out for each patient with a continence problem. It is a generic assessment, which applies equally to all patients, whatever their condition. Sign the box at the end of the CP. No other writing is necessary unless you wish to add comments. You should be aware, however, that when you sign the box you are stating that you have met all the standards contained within your section of the CP.

Information sheet 2

Medications affecting urinary continence status

Medication	Indication	Side effect
Alimemazine tartrate	Allergies, urticaria, pruritus	Difficulty with micturition, retention
Alprazolam	Anxiety	Retention, decreased awareness, incontinence
Alprostadil	Erectile dysfunction	Frequency, urgency, impaired urination
Amantadine hydrochloride	Influenza, Parkinson's disease	Incontinence, retention

Medication	Indication	Side effect
Amiloride hydrochloride	Hypertension, oedema congestive cardiac failure	Frequency and urgency
Amitriptyline	Depressive illness	Difficulty with micturition
Amlodipine besilate	Hypertension, angina prophylaxis	Frequency
Amoxapine	Depressive illness	Difficulty with micturition
Atropine sulfate	gastrointestinal spasm	Urgency
Baclofen	Muscle spasticity	Urinary incontinence, urinary retention
Benzatropine mesylate	Parkinson's disease	Urinary retention
Brompheniramine (constituent of cough linctus)	Allergies	Difficulty with micturition, retention
Buprenorphine	Pain	Difficulty with micturition
Carbidopa	Parkinson's disease	Incontinence, retention
Carmustine implant (Gliadel)	Glioma	Urinary tract infection, incontinence
Carvedilol	Chronic heart failure, hypertension, angina	Incontinence (in females)
Chlordiazepoxide	Anxiety	Retention, decreased awareness, incontinence
Chlorphenamine maleate	Allergies	Difficulty with micturition, retention
Chlorpromazine hydrochloride	Psychosis, mania, schizophrenia	Difficulty with micturition
Chlortalidone	Hypertension, oedema congestive cardiac failure, diabetes insipidus	Frequency and urgency

Medication	Indication	Side effect
Citalopram	Depressive illness, obsessive-compulsive disorder	Urinary retention
Clemastine	Allergies	Difficulty with micturition, retention
Clomipramine hydrochloride	Depressive illness, phobic states	Difficulty with micturition
Clonazepam	Epilepsy	Urinary incontinence
Clozapine	Schizophrenia	Difficulty with micturition
Cyclopenthiazide	Hypertension, oedema congestive cardiac failure	Frequency and urgency
Cyproheptadine hydrochloride	Allergies	Difficulty with micturition, retention
Dantrolene sodium	Muscle spasticity, malignant hyperthermia	Frequency, incontinence, retention
Darifenacin	Bladder instability	Retention of urine, bladder pain
Diazepam	Anxiety, insomnia, muscle spasm	Retention, decreased awareness, incontinence
Dicycloverine	Irritable bowel syndrome, gastrointestinal spasm	Urgency
Dihydrocodeine tartrate	Pain	Urinary retention
Diphenhydramine hydrochloride	Allergies	Difficulty with micturition, retention
Dipipanone	Pain	Difficulty with micturition
Disopyramide	Ventricular arrhythmias	Retention of urine

Medication	Indication	Side effect
Donepezil hydrochloride	Alzheimer's dementia	Urinary incontinence
Dosulepin hydrochloride	Depressive illness	Difficulty with micturition
Dothiepin hydrochloride	Depressive illness	Difficulty with micturition
Doxazosin	Hypertension	Incontinence
Doxepin	Depressive illness	Difficulty with micturition
Doxylamine	Cough, decongestant	Difficulty with micturition, retention
Etodolac	Osteo- and rheumatoid arthritis	Frequency, dysuria
Eletriptan	Migraine	Urinary frequency, polyuria
Ephedrine hydrochloride	Hypotension, nasal congestion	Retention, difficulty with micturition
Escitalopram	Depressive illness, obsessive-compulsive disorder	Urinary retention
Felodipine	Hypertension, angina prophylaxis	Frequency
Fentanyl	Breakthrough pain	Urinary retention
Flavoxate hydrochloride	Urinary frequency	Difficulty with micturition
Flurazepam	Insomnia	Retention, decreased awareness, incontinence
Frovatriptan	Migraine	Micturition frequency, polyuria
Gabapentin	Epilepsy	Incontinence
Galantamine	Alzheimer's dementia	Urinary tract infection
Hydroxyzine hydrochloride	Allergies, pruritus, anxiety	Difficulty with micturition, retention

Medication	Indication	Side effect
Hyoscine butylbromide	Diverticular disease	Urgency
Hyoscine hydrobromide	Motion sickness	Difficulty with micturition
Imipramine	Depressive illness	Difficulty with micturition
Indapamide	Hypertension, oedema congestive cardiac failure	Frequency and urgency
Indoramin	Hypertension	Urinary frequency, incontinence
Isocarboxazid	Depressive illness	Difficulty with micturition
Isoniazid	Pulmonary tuberculosis	Difficulty with micturition
Lacidipine	Hypertension, angina prophylaxis	Frequency
Levomepromazine	Schizophrenia	Difficulty with micturition
Lithium	Bipolar disorder, mania	Polyuria
Lofepramine	Depressive illness	Difficulty with micturition
Loprazolam	Insomnia, anxiety	Retention, decreased awareness, incontinence
Lorazepam	Anxiety, insomnia	Retention, decreased awareness, incontinence
Lormetazepam	Insomnia	Retention, decreased awareness, incontinence
Lumiracoxib	Osteoarthritis	Frequency
Maprotiline	Depressive illness	Difficulty with micturition
Meptazinol	Pain	Difficulty with micturition

Medication	Indication	Side effect
Methadone hydrochloride	Opioid dependence	Difficulty with micturition
Metolazone	Hypertension, oedema congestive cardiac failure	Frequency and urgency
Mianserin	Depressive illness	Difficulty with micturition
Morphine sulfate	Pain	Difficulty with micturition
Nalbuphine	Pain	Difficulty with micturition
Nicardipine hydrochloride	Hypertension, angina prophylaxis	Frequency
Nifedipine	Hypertension, angina prophylaxis, Reynaud's syndrome	Frequency
Nisoldipine	Hypertension, angina prophylaxis	Frequency
Nitrazepam	Insomnia	Retention, decreased awareness, incontinence
Nortriptyline	Depressive illness	Difficulty with micturition
Olanzapine hydrochloride	Schizophrenia	Urinary hesitation
Orphenadrine	Parkinson's disease	Urinary retention
Oxazepam	Anxiety	Retention, decreased awareness, incontinence
Oxybutynin hydrochloride	Bladder instability	Difficulty with micturition
Oxycodone hydrochloride	Pain	Urinary retention
Paliperidone	Schizophrenia	Urinary incontinence
Pentazocine	Pain	Difficulty with micturition

Medication	Indication	Side effect
Papaveretum	Pain	Difficulty with micturition
Periciazine	Schizophrenia and other psychoses	Difficulty with micturition
Phenelzine	Depressive illness	Difficulty with micturition
Pipotiazine palmitate	Schizophrenia	Difficulty with micturition
Prazosin	Hypertension, Reynaud's syndrome, congestive cardiac failure	Frequency, incontinence
Pregabalin	Neuropathic pain, epilepsy, generalised anxiety disorder	Urinary incontinence, dysuria
Procyclidine hydrochloride	Parkinson's disease	Urinary retention
Promazine	Agitation and restlessness	Difficulty with micturition
Promethazine hydrochloride	Allergies	Difficulty with micturition, retention
Propantheline bromide	gastrointestinal spasm	Urgency
Propiverine hydrochloride	Frequency, urgency	Difficulty with micturition
Rasagiline	Parkinson's disease	Urgency
Reboxetine	Depressive illness, anxiety	Urinary retention
Risperidone	Psychoses, mania	Incontinence
Solifenacin succinate	Frequency, urgency	Difficulty with micturition
Somatropin	Growth failure	Incontinence, frequency
Sulindac	Arthritis, inflammatory disorders	Dysuria

Medication	Indication	Side effect
Temazepam	Insomnia	Retention, decreased awareness, incontinence
Terazosin	Hypertension, benign prostatic hyperplasia	Frequency, incontinence
Tolterodine tartrate	Frequency urgency	Difficulty with micturition
Tranylcypromine	Depressive illness	Difficulty with micturition
Trazodone	Depressive illness	Difficulty with micturition
Triamterene	Hypertension, oedema congestive cardiac failure	Frequency, urgency
Trihexyphenidyl hydrochloride	Parkinson's disease	Urinary retention
Trimeprazine tartrate	Allergies	Difficulty with micturition, retention
Trimipramine	Depressive illness	Difficulty with micturition
Triprolidine	Cough, decongestant	Difficulty with micturition, retention
Trospium chloride	Frequency, urgency	Difficulty with micturition
Venlafaxine	Depressive illness, generalised anxiety disorder	Urinary frequency
Xipamide	Hypertension, oedema congestive cardiac failure	Frequency, urgency
Zolmitriptan	Migraine	Urinary frequency, polyuria

Information sheet 3

Medication which may be associated with constipation

Medication	Indication
Alendronic acid	Osteoporosis
Alfuzosin	Benign prostatic hypertrophy
Aluminium hydroxide	Digestive disorders
Amisulpride	Schizophrenia
Amitriptyline hydrochloride	Depression
Aprepitant	Nausea and vomiting
Beclometasone dipropionate	Mild to moderate ulcerative colitis, asthma, allergic and vasomotor rhinitis
Benperidol	Antipsychotic
Buprenorphine	Analgesia
Carbamazepine	Epilepsy
Chlorpromazine hydrochloride	Antipsychotic
Chlorpropamide	Diabetes
Citalopram	Depression
Clomipramine hydrochloride	Depression
Clonidine hydrochloride	Hypertension, migraine, menopausal flushing
Clozapine	Schizophrenia
Cocodamol	Pain
Codeine phosphate	Analgesia
Darifenacin	Urinary incontinence
Diamorphine hydrochloride	Analgesia
Dihydrocodeine tartrate	Analgesia
Dipipanone hydrochloride	Analgesia
Disodium etidronate	Osteoporosis
Dosulepin hydrochloride	Depression
Doxazosin	Benign prostatic hypertrophy

Medication	Indication
Duloxetine	Stress incontinence, urinary incontinence
Entacapone	Parkinson's disease
Escitalopram	Depression
Esomeprazole	Gastro-oesophageal reflux, gastric ulcer
Etodolac	Pain and inflammation of rheumatoid- and osteoarthritis
Fentanyl	Analgesia
Ferrous fumarate	Iron-deficiency anaemia
Ferrous gluconate	Iron-deficiency anaemia
Ferrous sulfate	Iron-deficiency anaemia
Fesoterodine	Urinary incontinence
Fluoxetine	Depression
Flupentixol	Antipsychotic
Fluvoxamine maleate	Depression
Frovatriptan	Migraine
Gabapentin	Epilepsy
Glibenclamide	Diabetes
Gliclazide	Diabetes
Glimepiride	Diabetes
Glucosamine	Osteoarthritis
Haloperidol	Antipsychotic
Hydromorphone Hydrochloride	Analgesia
Imipramine hydrochloride	Depression
Indoramin	Benign prostatic hypertrophy
Lansoprazole	Gastro-oesophageal reflux, gastric ulcer
Levofloxacin	Antibiotic
Levomepromazine	Antipsychotic
Lofepramine	Depression
Magnesium complexes	Digestive disorders
Mefenamic acid	Mild to moderate pain

Medication	Indication
Memantine hydrochloride	Alzheimer's dementia
Meptazinol	Analgesia
Methadone hydrochloride	Analgesia
Morphine salts	Analgesia
Moxifloxacin	Antibiotic
Nisoldipine	Angina, hypertension
Nortriptyline	Depression
Omeprazole	Gastro-oesophageal reflux, gastric ulcer
Oxcarbazepine	Epilepsy
Oxybutynin hydrochloride	Urinary incontinence
Oxycodone hydrochloride	Analgesia
Pantoprazole	Gastro-oesophageal reflux, gastric ulcer
Papaveretum	Analgesia
Parathyroid hormone	Osteoporosis
Paroxetine	Depression
Pentazocine	Analgesia
Pergolide	Parkinson's disease
Pericyazine	Antipsychotic
Perphenazine	Antipsychotic
Pethidine hydrochloride	Analgesia
Phenelzine	Depression
Phenytoin	Epilepsy
Pimozide	Antipsychotic
Piperacillin	Antibiotic
Pramipexole	Parkinson's disease
Prazosin	Benign prostatic hypertrophy
Pregabalin	Epilepsy
Prochlorperazine	Antipsychotic
Proguanil hydrochloride	Antimalarial
Promazine hydrochloride	Antipsychotic
Propafenone hydrochloride	Arrhythmia

Medication	Indication
Quetiapine	Schizophrenia
Rabeprazole sodium	Gastro-oesophageal reflux, gastric ulcer
Rasagiline	Parkinsonism
Reboxetine	Major depression
Repaglinide	Type II diabetes
Risedronate sodium	Osteoporosis
Rotigotine	Parkinson's disease
Rufinamide	Epilepsy
Rufinamide	Epilepsy
Selegiline hydrochloride	Parkinson's disease
Sertraline	Depression
Sibutramine hydrochloride	Obesity
Sucralfate	Gastritis
Sulpiride	Schizophrenia
Tamsulosin	Benign prostatic hypertrophy
Terazosin	Benign prostatic hypertrophy
Tolbutamide	Diabetes
Tolcapone	Parkinson's disease
Tolteradine tartrate	Urinary incontinence
Tramadol hydrochloride	Analgesia
Trifluoperazine	Antipsychotic
Trimipramine	Depression
Tripotassium dicitratobismuthate	Gastric and duodenal ulceration
Trospium chloride	Urinary incontinence
Venlafaxine	Depression
Verapamil hydrochloride	Angina hypertension
Zotepine	Antipsychotics
Zuclopenthixol acetate	Antipsychotic

Information sheet 4

Abdominal massage

Throughout the ages, therapeutic massage has been used to great effect in the healing environment. Abdominal massage as a therapy to relieve constipation has been known to be effective for many hundreds of years, but was given a higher profile in the 1870s by the American John Kellogg (inventor of Cornflakes). He recommended 'abdominal massage with a leather-coated cannon ball weighing three to four pounds for men with sluggish colons'.

In some spinal units and hospices massage around the abdomen is performed, and patients and carers are taught the technique. The aim of the massage is to release spasm in the abdomen to allow normal gut activity and increase peristalsis.

Contraindications for the use of abdominal massage are cancer of the bowel, herniation of the abdomen, recent surgery or scarring. Patients on anticoagulants should be treated with caution, as massage may induce bleeding.

There should be an initial assessment which should include:

- GP consent
- informed consent of the patient
- medical history of constipation over past six months
- frequency of enemas
- medication taken
- daily food and fluid intake
- degree of mobility
- physical problems
- access to toilet facilities
- psychological problems.

By monitoring massage and bowel movement over a period of four to six weeks, effectiveness can be evaluated. Once a pattern has been established, patients can be taught to self-massage or carers can be trained.

Massage procedure

Grapeseed oil or baby oil is used to make the massage as smooth and comfortable as possible.

- Place a rolled towel or pillow under the knees to relax the abdomen.
- Stroke abdominal wall gently downwards from stomach to groin with one hand following the other alternately.
- When you feel the muscles relax, effleurage (strong stroke which makes firm contact of the whole hand with the body as it moves slowly along) is carried out along the line of the colon, beginning in the right iliac fossa and travelling along the ascending, transverse and descending colon.
- After several effleurage strokes, circular kneading along the line of the colon, moving in the same direction as before. This is a fairly slow, fairly deep movement performed with the whole of the hand.
- Repeat the effleurage strokes and complete the massage by side-to-side stroking across the abdominal wall.
- Massage for 15–20 minutes.

Information sheet 5

Laxatives

The ideal management of constipation involves the identification and, if possible, elimination of the primary cause, education of the patient in the physiology of defecation, initiation of a proper diet and prescription of appropriate laxatives until bowel function is restored.

Laxatives used in constipation can be classified into the five groups listed below and outlined in the table at the end of this information sheet.

Bulking agents (e.g. bran, sterculia, isphagula)

The agents absorb water and expand to fill the colon with soft, non-absorbable residue and appear to have few side effects. Caution is advised in using bulking agents with older patients, as this may lead to severe dehydration.

Mild constipation may respond to simple dietary manipulation, which can be useful in prophylaxis, but use doubtful if constipation bad enough to seek help. The aim is to increase bulk and therefore to reduce transit time, propelling a softer stool into the rectum. Needs to be combined with minor lifestyle changes, including allowing adequate time for defecation and not ignoring the call to stool.

To avoid bloating/abdominal pain, fibre should be increased gradually. Avoid fibre supplements in older patients, as they may cause faecal incontinence.

Finding a laxative that works for the individual is trial and error. Try bulking agents for those who find dietary fibre supplements unpalatable. These must be introduced gradually. Use after clearance of impacted faeces and adequate fluids, or there will be a danger of intestinal obstruction or adding to faecal mass.

Most commonly used to treat chronic dystonic or spastic constipation. Dietary/bulking agents will exacerbate faecal impaction. Bulk-forming agents may inhibit the patient's appetite and contribute to malnourishment. High bran intake has been linked with impaired calcium/iron reabsorption. These agents need to be taken over several days to take effect, and should be accompanied by raised fluid intake to prevent impaction/obstruction. The most commonly used are Normacol and Fybogel; they are useful in the management of patients with haemorrhoids and anal fissures. These products swell on contact with water and therefore must not be used for dysphagic patients or immediately prior to going to bed.

It is suggested that better effects may be obtained from bulk-forming laxatives that can be incorporated into the diet, for example wholegrain cereals and high-fibre bread. Increased fluid intake is required, especially for older patients. However, they do tend to distend the abdomen initially, making the patient feel uncomfortable, and this can lead to temporary anorexia. Bran is cheap, but care is needed – as above.

Glycerine suppositories can be used in addition to bulk-forming laxatives for simple constipation.

Hyper-osmotic laxatives

These are divided into inorganic and organic osmotic agents.

Inorganic agents (e.g. preparations that contain magnesium or sulfate salts or both).

For many years these agents have been thought to act simply as osmotic laxatives by softening and increasing water absorption in the stool, but the rapidity and potency of their effect have led to a pharmacological re-evaluation. This has shown that they act both directly and through the release of cholecystokinin to cause contraction of the gall bladder, increased motility of the small and large intestine, decreased absorption of sodium by the small intestinal mucosa and increased secretion of pancreatic enzymes. The osmotic load that they deliver causes large losses of faecal water and consequent electrolyte disturbances that can be serious if cardiac function is impaired.

Organic agents (e.g. lactulose)

These are non-absorbable solutes that act by softening and increasing water absorption, such as lactulose. Lactulose is metabolised by the colonic bacterial flora to produce short-chain fatty acids, and its laxative effect is associated with a marked production of gases, including carbon dioxide, methane and hydrogen. Most of the common side effects attributed to lactulose – such as abdominal pain, bloating and flatus – are thought to result from this colonic fermentation. The capacity of gut bacteria for lactulose is limited, so that above a certain dose, if constipation is not relieved, there is no further benefit in giving additional lactulose to the patient. These agents may take up to 48 hours to act, and bloating, flatulence, cramping and an unpleasant taste have all been reported.

Lactulose is generally not suitable for the prevention of constipation where gut motility is impaired, for example with anticholinergic and opioid treatment unless accompanied by stimulants, such as senna. Lactulose takes one to three days to act and may cause flatulence, cramps and bloating. It is suitable for chronic constipation where the stool is hard.

Other information

Most opioid-induced constipation requires a combination of stimulant and softener. Dose titrated to comfort of defecation and nature of stool. For older people with chronic constipation, treatment with laxatives is essential. Stimulant could be used short term if constipation persists. Bulk-forming agent could be added. If this is unsuccessful, use iso-osmotic agent.

Iso-osmotic agents (e.g. macrogol)

These consist of an organic, non-absorbable solute such as polyethylene glycol (PEG) balanced with electrolytes. This balanced solution induces an osmotic load while achieving negligible net absorption or elimination of water, sodium or potassium. Potentially serious losses or gains in water and electrolytes are prevented. PEG is also free from the potential toxicity of stimulant laxatives. Thus, the solution remains in the colon, where it increases the faecal bulk, causing stretching of the circular muscle in the bowel wall and triggering myogenic peristalsis movement. The liquid is also available to soften and lubricate the faecal residue. Thus, the stools are rehydrated and softened and comfortable bowel emptying is facilitated.

Iso-osmotic treatments are significantly different from other osmotic laxatives as their effect is not via a hyper-osmotic action, pulling fluid and electrolytes into the colon from the bloodstream, but essentially by retaining within the bowel, fluid and electrolytes ingested along with the osmotically active component PEG.

Stool softeners (e.g. liquid paraffin, docusate)

These are helpful in selected groups of patients such as those with cardiac impairment, because they reduce straining at defecation.

These act by reducing surface tension, allowing penetration of hardened faeces by water/fats. The group includes mineral oil and docusate salts, which also act as a stimulant. Liquid paraffin is not recommended for oral use as it inhibits absorption of fat-soluble vitamins. If aspirated, it may cause lipid pneumonia. They act in 24–48 hours.

Stimulant laxatives (e.g. senna, bisacodyl)

Stimulant laxatives increase intestinal motility by stimulation of colonic nerves and may cause abdominal cramping. If used repeatedly, these agents can cause irreversible damage to myenteric neurons. In experimental studies their hydroxylated metabolites have been found to be mutagenic and carcinogenic.

Prolonged or over dosage of stimulants can result in diarrhoea, with excessive water loss with electrolytes (especially potassium), which may lead to an atonic, non-functioning colon. They should not be given to patients with faecal impaction, intestinal obstruction or undiagnosed abdominal symptoms. They can irritate the mucosa, nerves and smooth muscle, producing cramping, electrolyte imbalance, histological changes and eventually permanent damage to the mesenteric plexus.

Eventually permanent damage affecting motility of gut = patient takes more drug.

Sodium picosulfate has a very dramatic effect and is reserved for bowel preparation. It must be used with extreme caution if there is suspicion of faecal impaction, especially in older patients or those with concurrent disease (diverticulitis).

Anthraquinones (senna, cascara, danthron, bisacodyl, castor oil and glycerine) may have adverse reactions, such as cramping, nausea, vomiting, diarrhoea and in some cases dehydration. They may discolour the urine from pink to red or brown to black as a result of elimination of metabolites and may discolour the colonic mucosa.

Senna is the most powerful. It has an effective, short-term use for acute constipation, usually within six to 12 hours, and is best given at bedtime. Demonstrated as an effective counteragent for opioids, as it reverses the alteration of colonic motility without reducing any analgesic effect. It is effective and relatively safe for older patients.

Bisacodyl can be administered either orally or rectally; if oral, it should be swallowed whole to avoid impairment of enteric coating. Its oral toxicity is low. The suppository is effective within 15 to 60 minutes. It is important that it make contact with the rectal wall when given to be effective. They may cause irritation or epithelial sloughing, so caution with patients with haemorrhoids or anal fissures must be urged.

Glycerine suppositories act as a bowel stimulant and stool softener.

Rectal preparations (e.g. arachis oil, docusate sodium, glycerine)

These preparations include enemas, micro-enemas and suppositories, which provide rapid relief from constipation. They can be combinations of both osmotic and stimulant laxatives and come in a number of different sizes, ranging from small 5 ml micro-enemas up to large 133 ml phosphate enemas – long-term use not recommended.

Laxative classes and examples

Laxative class	Example
Bulk	Bran Sterculia Ispaghula husk Methylcellulose
Hyper-osmotic	Magnesium carbonate Magnesium hydroxide Magnesium sulfate Lactulose
Iso-osmotic	Polyethylene glycol + electrolytes
Stool softeners	Docusate Liquid paraffin
Stimulant	Anthraquinones: ● Senna ● Cascara ● Danthron Diphenyl methane derivatives: ● Bisacodyl ● Sodium picosulfate
Rectal preparations	● Docusate ● Glycerine

Information sheet 6

Autonomic dysreflexia

Autonomic dysreflexia is seen particularly in patients with cervical injuries above the sympathetic outflow but may occur in those with high thoracic lesions above T6. It may occur at any time after the period of spinal shock and is most commonly caused by a distended bladder but may be caused by other conditions which cause visceral stimulation, for example infection, loaded colon, anal fissure, ejaculation during intercourse and labour.

The effect is that there is reflex sympathetic overactivity below the level of the spinal cord lesion, causing vasoconstriction and systemic hypertension. The carotid and aortic baroreceptors are stimulated and respond via the vasomotor centre with increased vagal tone and resulting bradycardia; but the peripheral vasodilation which would normally have relieved the hypertension does not occur, as stimuli cannot pass distally through the injured cord.

Symptoms of autonomic dysreflexia are, characteristically, pounding headache, profuse sweating, flushing or blotchiness above the level of the lesion. Without prompt treatment, intercranial haemorrhage may occur.

Treatment consists of removing the precipitating cause. If hypertension persists, prescribe 5–10 mg nifedipine or 250 μg glyceryl trinitrate sublingually, or 5–10 mg phentolamine intravenously

If inadequately treated, the patient can become sensitised and develop repeated attacks with minimal stimuli.

Occasionally, sympathetic activity may need to be blocked by spinal or epidural anaesthesia.

Information sheet 7

Neurogenic bowel management

A neurogenic bowel is a life-altering impairment of gastrointestinal and anorectal function resulting from a lesion of the nervous system, commonly following spinal cord injury (SCI). Research has showed a high prevalence of gastrointestinal complaints and a negative impact on daily living after SCI. Among the complications and evacuation problems are ileus, gastric ulcers, gastro-oesophageal reflux, autonomic dysreflexia, pain, abdominal distension, diverticulosis, haemorrhoids, nausea, loss of appetite, constipation, impaction, diarrhoea and delayed or unplanned evacuation.

Anatomy and physiology

Continence

In the normal bowel, continence is maintained by a combination of the actions of the internal anal sphincter (IAS) and the puborectalis muscle. In the resting state, faecal continence is maintained by a closed IAS and by the acute angle of the anorectal canal produced by the puborectalis sling. IAS tone is inhibited with rectal dilatation by stool or digital stimulation. Reflex contraction of the external anal sphincter (EAS) and the puborectalis prevents incontinence with cough or Valsalva manoeuvre. Voluntary control of abdominal musculature and relaxation of the EAS permit wilful defecation at times of increased colonic motility.

Innervation

The bowel is extrinsically innervated by sympathetic, parasympathetic and somatic nerves. The colon wall contains an enteric nervous system, which coordinates much of its movement. Reflex pathways from the central nervous system to the intestine and colon both facilitate and inhibit motility.

Gastrocolic reflex

The gastrocolic reflex, triggered by feeding, produces propulsive peristalsis of the small intestine and colon. The precise mechanism has not been conclusively defined, and studies with individuals following SCI have shown conflicting results. It is suggested that the gastrocolic reflex remains intact in many people with SCI.

Information sheet 8

Neurogenic bowel responses

Depending on the location of the injury, spinal cord injury (SCI) produces two different patterns of bowel dysfunction.

An injury above the sacral segments produces an upper motor neuron (UMN) bowel in which defecation cannot be initiated by voluntary relaxation of the external anal sphincter (EAS). Inability to voluntarily modulate descending inhibition and spasticity of the pelvic floor prevents EAS relaxation, thus promoting stool retention. However, nerve connections between the spinal cord and the colon and in the colonic wall remain intact, permitting reflex coordination of stool propulsion.

Complete injury at the sacral segments (or the cauda equina) results in an areflexic or lower motor neuron (LMN) bowel in which no spinal cord mediated reflex peristalsis occurs. The myenteric plexus within the colonic wall coordinates slow stool movement, a dryer, rounder shape and a greater risk of faecal incontinence through the hypotonic anal sphincter.

Difficulties with evacuation include:

- delayed or painful evacuation
- constipation
- hard, round stools that may be difficult to evacuate
- diarrhoea
- unplanned evacuations occurring between planned bowel care.

Individuals with UMN SCI will usually require the insertion of suppositories (glycerine or bisacodyl) and/or digital anal stimulation to initiate defecation. Stimulant laxatives should be avoided, as prolonged use may lead to an atonic bowel and exacerbate evacuation difficulties. Enemas should not be used, owing to the risk of injury to the anus/rectal mucosa or of perforation of the bowel with symptoms masked by the SCI. The amount of assistance required will be affected by the level of the injury and by other factors, such as age and cognitive ability. An upright position provides the most rapid and effective evacuation, but risk factors of this position must be considered.

Information sheet 9

Normal bowel habits

The bowel has five main functions:

1. **Storage:** The colon stores unabsorbed food residue. Within 72 hours of intake, 70% of food residue has been excreted. The remaining 30% stays in the colon for up to a week or more. The longer food residue remains in the colon, the more water is reabsorbed and the harder the stools produced become.
2. **Absorption:** Sodium, water, chloride and some fat-soluble vitamins are all absorbed from the colon. Some drugs, for example some steroids and aspirin, are also absorbed by the colonic mucous membrane.

3. **Secretion:** Mucus is secreted by the colon to lubricate the faeces and aid expulsion.
4. **Synthesis of some vitamins:** Bacteria which colonize the colon are responsible for the production of small amounts of vitamin K, thiamine, folic acid and riboflavin.
5. **Elimination:** The main function of the colon is the propulsion of faecal matter and the absorption of fluid.

Normal control of defecation

1. When faeces enter the rectum, their presence is detected by sensory nerve endings in the muscle around the rectum. This results in a sensation of rectal fullness, and the desire to defecate.
2. Defecation involves the relaxation of two sphincters: the internal anal sphincter (under autonomic control) and the external anal sphincter (under both autonomic and voluntary control).
3. A volume of about 150 ml of faeces causes autonomic relaxation of the internal anal sphincter.
4. Faeces then enter the anal canal. Sensitive nerve endings relay messages to the brain, which are interpreted as urgency. Very sensitive squamous epithelium can distinguish between gas, fluid and solid matter entering the canal, even during sleep.
5. If it is convenient to defecate, the external sphincter relaxes. A reflex action from the spinal cord will initiate defecation. In adults this can be inhibited by the cerebral cortex if defecation is inconvenient, thereby giving the patient control over this mechanism.
6. The stool is then expelled by rectal contraction. The position of the body is also important, as gravity and the abdominal effort (straining) aid expulsion.
7. Unless the stool is hard (owing to constipation), only a small amount of abdominal effort is required to propel the stool through the anal canal.
8. Any injury or disease which interferes with this mechanism (for example pelvic floor damage following childbirth) can result in constipation.

Maintenance of continence

There are two key mechanisms:

1. The external anal sphincter: this maintains a continuous resting muscular tone, which can be greatly augmented by voluntary or involuntary muscular contraction over short periods.
   (a) Voluntary contraction can be used to inhibit the reflex. If the rectum is full and the internal sphincter has relaxed, but for social reasons defecation is not desirable, contraction of the external sphincter will force the faeces up into the rectum. This mechanism also allows the retention of liquid diarrhoea or flatus.
   (b) Involuntary reflex contraction of the external anal sphincter can be stimulated by increases in intro-abdominal pressure.
2. The anorectal angle: the puborectalis muscle sling of the pelvic floor helps to maintain a right angle between the anus and rectum, which acts as a barrier to the movement of faeces. When abdominal pressure is raised, reflex contraction of the pelvic floor helps maintain the anorectal angle and prevents the faeces being propelled from the rectum to the anus.

Information sheet 10

Bowel diary

Date and time	Bristol Stool type	Incontinent episodes	Any other comments (e.g. laxatives, cause, diet)

Information sheet 11

Symptoms and causes of obstruction

	Small bowel	Large bowel	Paralytic ileus	Strangulated obstruction
History				
Surgical	Adhesions from previous abdominal surgery		Recent abdominal surgery	Previous surgery or adhesions
Medical	Hernia, shock, occlusion of mesenteric arteries, radiation, gall stone migration	Tumour, diverticulitis, volvulus, intussusception, ulcerative colitis, mesenteric occlusion, faecal impaction, radiation	Pneumonia, pancreatitis, kidney infection, spinal cord injury, diabetic ketoacidosis, hypokalaemia, bile irritation	Any type of obstruction can progress to the point where the bowel contorts and cuts off blood supply
Drugs	Cardiac glycosides, diuretics, opiates, anticholinergics, tricyclic antidepressants	Cardiac glycosides, diuretics, opiates, anticholinergics, tricyclic antidepressants	Cardiac glycosides, diuretics, opiates, anticholinergics, tricyclic antidepressants	Cardiac glycosides, diuretics, opiates, anticholinergics, tricyclic antidepressants

Symptoms

Onset	Rapid	Insidious	As early as 1–2 days post-operatively or as late as 6 weeks post op	Rapid
Vomiting	Early and frequent if high up, with lower blockage later and may contain faeces	Secondary to distension of small intestine; late onset may contain faeces	Usually not prominent, may only follow eating	Early: infrequent Late: persistent
Pain	Cramping in mid- to upper abdomen, episodic increases after meals, can be severe	Moderate cramping in suprapubic area	Dull, diffuse, continuous	Severe cramping in mid-epigastric/periumbilical area

Signs

Abdomen	Non-tender, distension occurs in later stages	Distension in later stages	Distension; tense shiny skin	Distension, rigidity
Bowel sounds	Early: high-pitched tinkling Intermittent Later: decreased or absent	Early: high-pitched tinkling Intermittent Later: decreased or absent	Infrequent or absent	Infrequent or absent

Information sheet 12

Constipation: signs and symptoms

Symptom	Visit 1	Visit 2	Visit 3
Do you have to make an effort and strain to pass bowel motion?			
Do you feel that your bowel motions are not frequent/regular enough? How often do you go and how often would you like to go?			
Do you have any pain or discomfort? State where, when and how much.			
Do you have the feeling that your bowel is not empty or you need to go again quickly?			
Stool chart score Any other comments			

References

Abrams, P., Cardozo, L., Fall, M. *et al.* (2002) The standardization of terminology of lower urinary tract function: Report from the Standardization Sub Committee of the International Continence Society. *Neurourology and Urodynamics* **21**, 167–178.

Addison, R. and Smith, M. (1995) *Digital rectal examination and manual removal of faeces*, Royal College of Nursing, London.

Anders, R.L., Tomai, J.S., Clute, R.M. and Olson, T. (1997) Development of a scientifically valid co-ordinated care path. *Journal of Nursing Administration* **27** (5), 45–52.

Anon (2004) A critical review of caffeine withdrawal: empirical validation of symptoms and signs, incidence, severity and associated features. *Psychopharmacology* **176** (1), 1–29.

Arnaud, M.J. (2003) Mild dehydration: A risk factor for constipation? *European Journal of Clinical Nutrition* **57** (suppl. 2), 88–95.

Audit Commission (1999) *First Assessment: A review of District Nursing Services in England and Wales*, Audit Commission, London.

Avery, K., Donovan, J., Peters, T.J. *et al.* (2004) ICIQ: a brief and robust measure for evaluating the symptoms and impact of urinary incontinence. *Neurourology & Urodynamics* **23** (4), 322–30.

Avorn, J., Monane, M., Gurwitz, J.H. *et al.* (1994) Reduction of bacteriuria and pyuria after ingestion of cranberry juice. *Journal of the American Medical Association* **271** (10), 751–754.

Ayas, S., Leblebici, B., Sozay, S. *et al.* (2006) The effect of abdominal massage on bowel function in patients with spinal cord injury. *American Journal of Physical Medicine and Rehabilitation* **85** (12), 951–955.

Bardsley, A. (2000) The neurogenic bladder. *Nursing Standard* **14** (22), 39–41.

Bayliss, V., Cherry, M., Locke, R. and Salter, L. (2000) Pathways for continence care: background and audit. *British Journal of Nursing* **9** (9), 590–596.

Bayliss, V., Cherry, M., Locke, R. and Salter, L. (2000a) Pathways for continence care: development of the pathways. *British Journal of Nursing* **9** (17), 1165–1172.

Bayliss, V., Salter, L. and Locke, R. (2001) Pathways for continence care: the validation process. *British Journal of Nursing* **10** (2), 87–90.

Bayliss, V., Salter, L. and Locke, R. (2003) Pathways for continence care: an audit to assess how they are used. *British Journal of Nursing* **12** (14), 857–863.

BBC Radio 4 (2005) *The Expert Patient*, Radio 4, Thursday 4th August, 8 p.m. to 8.30 p.m., http://www.bbc.co.uk/radio4/science/expertpatient.shtml).

Berghmans, L.C., Hendriks, H.J., Bo, K. *et al.* (1998) Conservative treatment of stress urinary incontinence in women: a systematic review of randomized clinical trials. *British Journal of Urology* **82** (2), 181–191.

Bourcier, A., McGuire, E. and Abrams, P. (2004) *Pelvic Floor Disorders*, Elsevier Saunders, Philadelphia.

Cardozo, L., Robinson, D. and Miles, A. (2006) *The Effective Management of Stress Urinary Incontinence*, Aesculapius Medical Press, London.

Cartmail, G. (2006) Our health, our care, our say. *Community Practitioner* **79** (4) 108–109.

Castelo-Branco, C., Cancelo, M.J., Villero, J. *et al.* (2005) Management of post-menopausal vaginal atrophy and atrophic vaginitis. *Maturitas* **52** (suppl. 1), S46–52.

Chief Nursing Officer (1977) Standards of Nursing Care: Promotion of Continence and Management of Incontinence, CNO (SNC) 77.

Clarke, A., Allen, P., Anderson, S. *et al.* (eds) (2004) *Studying the Organisation and Delivery of Health Services: A Reader*, Routledge, London.

Coulter, A., Entwhistle, V. and Gilbert, D. (1998) *Informing Patients: An Assessment of the Quality of Patient Information Materials*, King's Fund, London.

De Luc, K. and Todd, J. (eds) (2003) *E-Pathways: Computers and the Patient's Journey Through Care*, Radcliffe Publishing, Abingdon.

Department of Health (1997) *The New NHS: Modern and Dependable*, HMSO, London.

Department of Health (1998) *A First Class Service: Quality in the New NHS*, HMSO, London.

Department of Health (1999) *Patient and Public Involvement in the NHS*, HMSO, London.

Department of Health (2000) *Good Practice in Continence Services*, HMSO, London.

Department of Health (2000a) *The NHS Plan*, HMSO, London.

Department of Health (2001) *Essence of Care*, HMSO, London.

Department of Health (2001a) *National Service Framework for Older People*, HMSO, London.

Department of Health (2003) *The NHS Patient Survey Programme*, HMSO, London.

Department of Health (2004) *NHS Improvement Plan*, London HMSO, London.

Department of Health (2006) *The NHS in England: The operating framework for 2007/08*, Department of Health, London.

Department of Health (2006a) *Our Health, Our Care, Our Say: A New Direction for Community Services*, Department of Health, London.

Department of Heath (2007) *Keeping it Personal: Clinical Case for Change*, HMSO, London.

Department of Health (2008) *NHS Next Stage Review: Our vision for Primary and Community Care*, HMSO, London.

Dolman, M. (1998) Strategies to promote continence in the community. *British Journal of Community Nursing* 33 (8), 385–392.

DuBeau, C.E., Levy, B., Mangione, C.M. and Resnick, N.M. (1998) The impact of urge urinary incontinence on quality of life: importance of patients' perspective and explanatory style. *Journal of the American Geriatrics Society* 46 (6), 683–692.

Duman, M. (2003) *The PoPPi Guide: Producing Patient Information*, King's Fund, London.

Dunn, N. (2003) Practical issues around putting the patients at the centre of care. *Journal of the Royal Society of Medicine* 96, 325–327.

Gask, L. and Usherwood, T. (2002) The consultation. *British Medical Journal* 324 (7353), 1567–1569.

Getliffe, K. and Dolman, M. (2003) *Promoting Continence*, Bailliere Tindall, London.

Ginsberg, D.A., Wallace, J., Phillips, S. and Josephson, K.L. (2007) Evaluating and managing constipation in the elderly. *Urologic Nursing* **27** (3), 191–200.

Godfrey, H. and Hogg, A. (2007) *Incontinence and Older People: Is there a link to social isolation?* Help the Aged, London.

Grundy, D. and Swain, A. (1996) *ABC of Spinal Cord Injury*, (3rd edn), BMJ Publishing, London.

Hay-Smith, E.J.C. and Dumoulin, C. (2006) Pelvic floor muscle training versus no treatment, or inactive control treatments, for urinary incontinence in women. *Cochrane Database of Systematic Reviews*, Issue 1. Art. No.: CD005654. DOI: 10.1002/14651858. CD005654.

Henwood, S. and Lister, J. (2007) *NLP and Coaching for Healthcare Professionals*, John Wiley & Sons, Ltd, Chichester.

Howell, A.B., Vorsa, N., Der Marderosian, A. and Foo, L.Y. (1998) Inhibition of the adherence of P-fimbriated Escherichia coli to uroepithelial-cell surfaces by proanthocyanidin extracts from cranberries. *New England Journal of Medicine* **339** (15), 1085–1086.

Hutchinson, S., Leger-Krall, S., Wilson, H.S. (1996) Toileting: a biobehavioral challenge in Alzheimer's dementia care. *Journal of Gerontological Nursing* **22** (10), 18–27.

Jepson, R.G. and Craig, J.C. (2008) Cranberries for preventing urinary tract infections. *Cochrane Database of Systematic Reviews* **1**, Art. No.: CD001321. DOI: 10.1002/14651858.CD001321.pub4.

Johnson, S. (ed) (1997) *Pathways of Care*, Blackwell Science, Oxford.

Jones, T. and Coyne, H. (2001) Modernisation and Care Pathways, The Association of Chartered Certified Accountants, London, http://www.acca.org.uk/pubs/members/publications/sector_booklets/healthcare_sector/care_pathway_booklet_2001.pdf, accessed 9 January 2009.

Juliano, L.M. and Griffiths, R.R. (2004) A critical review of caffeine withdrawal: empirical validation of symptoms and signs, incidence, severity and associated features. *Psychopharmacology* **176** (1), 1–29.

Kent, P. and Chalmers, Y. (2006) A decade on: Has the use of integrated pathways made a difference in Lanarkshire? *Journal of Nursing Management* **14** (7), 508–520.

Kitchiner, D. (1997) Analysis of Variation from the Pathway, in S. Johnson, (ed.), *Pathways of Care*, Blackwell, Oxford.

Kmietowicz, Z. (2006) UK Government to shift NHS power to community health care. *British Medical Journal* **332** (7536), 253.

Kohler-Ockmore, J. and Feneley, R. (1996) Long-term catheterisation of the bladder: prevalence and morbidity. *British Journal of Urology* **77**, 347–351.

Laycock, J. and Haslam, J. (eds) (2002) *Therapeutic Management of Incontinence and Pelvic Pain*, Springer-Verlag, London.

Leaver R.B. (1996) Cranberry juice. *Professional Nurse* **11** (8), 525–526.

Lesser, J., Hughes, B., Jemelka, J. and Kumar, M. (2005) Challenges and strategies for taking a comprehensive history in the elderly. *Geriatrics* **60** (11), 22–25.

Little, P., Everitt, H., Williamson, I. *et al.* (2001) Preferences of patients for patient centred approach to consultation in primary care: observational study. *British Medical Journal* **322** (7284), 468–472.

Lynn, M.R. (1986) Determination and quantification of content validity. *Nursing Research* **35** (6), 382–386.

Mandelstam, D. (1989) *Understanding Incontinence: A Guide to the Nature and Management of a Very Common Complaint*, Chapman & Hall, London.

Marcell, D., Ransel, S. and Schiau, M. (2003) Treatment Options Alleviate Female Urge Incontinence. *Nurse Practitioner* **28** (2), 48–55.

Martin, J.L., Williams, K.S., Abrams, K.R. *et al.* (2006) Systematic review and evaluation of methods of assessing urinary incontinence. *Health Technology Assessment* **10** (6), 1–132.

McKibbon, K.A. (1998) Evidence based practice. *Bulletin of the Medical Library Association* **86** (3), 396–401.

McNeill, P. (1990) *Research Methods*, Routledge, London.

Middleton, S. and Roberts, A. (2000) *Integrated Care Pathways: A Practical Approach to Implementation*, Butterworth Heinemann, Edinburgh.

Moehrer, B., Hextall, A. and Jackson, S. (2003) Oestrogens for urinary incontinence in women. *Cochrane Database of Systematic Reviews*, Issue 2. Art. No.: CD001405. DOI: 10.1002/14651858. CD001405.

National Institute for Health and Clinical Excellence (2006) *Urinary Incontinence: The Management of Urinary Incontinence in Women*, NICE Guideline 40, NICE, London.

National Institute for Health and Clinical Excellence (2007) *Faecal Incontinence. The Management of Faecal Incontinence in Adults*, NICE, London.

NHS Institute for Innovation and Improvement (2005) *Improvement Leaders' Guide: Process mapping, Analysis and Redesign*, NHS Institute for Innovation and Improvement, Coventry.

NHS Institute for Innovation and Improvement (2005a) *Improvement Leaders' Guide: Involving Patients and Carers. General improvement skills*, NHS Institute for Innovation and Improvement, Coventry.

Norton, C. (ed) (1996) *Nursing for Continence*, (2nd edn), Beaconsfield Publishers, Beaconsfield.

Norton, C. and Chelvanayagam, S. (eds) (2004) *Bowel Continence Nursing*, Beaconsfield Publishers, Beaconsfield.

O'Connor, J. and Lages, A. (2004) *Coaching with NLP*, Harper Collins, London.

O'Donnell, M. and Entwistle, V. (2003) *Producing Information about Health and Health Care Interventions: A practical guide*, University of Aberdeen, Aberdeen, http://www.abdn.ac.uk/hsru/pdf/revisedguide_090603.pdf, accessed 13 January 2009.

Parsons, M. and Cardozo, L. (2004) *Female Urinary Incontinence in Practice*, Royal Society of Medicine Press, London.

Pountney, D. (2008) £13bn cost for European economic burden of incontinence. *Nursing Older People* **20** (4), 4.

Rees, G., Huby, G., McDade, L. and McKechnie, L. (2004) Joint working in community mental health teams: implementation of an integrated care pathway. *Health & Social Care in the Community* **12** (6), 527–536.

Resende, T.L., Brocklehurst, J. and O'Neill, P.A. (1993) A pilot study on the effects of exercise and abdominal massage on bowel habit in continuing care patients. *Clinical Rehabilitation* **7**, 204–209.

Richards, S. (2008) Urinary tract infection. *Practice Nurse* **35** (11), 16–18.

Roberts, L. and Bucksey, S. (2007) Communicating with patients. *Physical Therapy* **87** (5), 586–594.

Robson, C. (1993) *Real World Research*, Blackwell, Oxford.

Rodgers, A., Bower, P., Gardner, C. *et al.* (2006) *The National Evaluation of the Pilot Phase of the Expert Patient Programme: Final*

Report, National Primary Care Research & Development Centre, University of Manchester/University of York, http://www.npcrdc. ac.uk/Publications/National_Evaluation_of_EPP_Report_2006. pdf, accessed 9 January 2009.

Roe, B. (1992) *Clinical Nursing Practice: The Promotion and Management of Continence*, Prentice Hall International, London.

Royal College of Nursing (2007) The RCN in history. *RCN Magazine* Spring, 6–7.

Royal College of Nursing (2008) *Bowel Care Including Digital Rectal Examination and the Manual Removal of Faeces*, RCN, London.

Royal College of Nursing Institute (1998) *Directory of NHS Trusts Using Care Pathways*, RCN, London.

Royal College of Physicians (1995) *Incontinence Causes, Management and Provision of Services*, RCP, London.

Sackett, D.L., Rosenberg, W.M., Gray, J.A. *et al.* (1996) Evidence based medicine: what it is and what it isn't. *British Medical Journal* **312** (7023), 71–72.

Scottish Intercollegiate Guidelines Network (2004) *Management of urinary incontinence in primary care: a national clinical guideline*, Royal College of Physicians, Edinburgh.

Shatell, M. and Hogan, B. (2005) Facilitating communication. *Journal of Psychosocial Nursing and Mental Health Service* **43** (10) 29–32.

Smith, E. and Ross, F. (2004) *Patient Experiences of Care Pathways: Cataract, Hip Replacement and Knee Arthroscopy: A Review of the Literature for the Commission for Health Improvement: Nurse Research Unit Report*, King's College, London.

Srikrishna, S., Robinson, D., Cardozo, L. and Vella, M. (2007) Management of overactive bladder syndrome. *Postgraduate Medical Journal* **83**, 481–486, doi: 10.1136/pgmj.2007.057232.

Starfield, B., Wray, C., Hess, K. *et al.* (1981) The influence of patient practitioner agreement on outcome of care. *American Journal of Public Health* **71** (2), 127.

Stavric, B., Klassen, R., Watkinson, B. *et al.* (1988) Variability in caffeine consumption from coffee and tea: Possible significance for epidemiological studies. *Foundations of Chemical Toxicology* **26** (2), 111–118.

Sulch, D., Melbourn, A., Perez, I. and Kalra, L. (2002) Integrated care pathways and quality of life on a stroke rehabilitation unit. *Stroke* **33** (6), 1600–1604.

Swami, S.K. and Abrams, P. (1996) Urge incontinence. *The Urologic Clinics of North America* **23** (3), 417–425.

Thomas, S. (2007) *Is Policy Translated into Action?*, RCN/ Continence Foundation, London.

Thomas, T.M., Plymat, K.R., Blannin, J. and Meade, T.W. (1980) Prevalence of urinary incontinence. *British Medical Journal* **281** (6250), 1243–5.

Thompson, W.G., Longstreth, G.F., Drossman, D.A. *et al.* (1999) Functional bowel disorders and functional abdominal pain. *GUT* **45** (suppl. 2), 1143–1147.

Timmins, N. (ed.) (2006) *Designing the New NHS: Ideas to Make a Supplier Market in Health Care Work*, King's Fund, London, http://www.kingsfund.org.uk/publications/kings_fund_publications/designing_the.html, accessed 9 January 2009.

Wagg, A. (2004) Urinary incontinence in older people: where are we now? *International Journal of Obstetrics & Gynaecology* **111** (suppl. 1), 15–19.

Wagg, A., Mian, S., Lowe, D. and Potter, J. (2005) *National Audit of Continence Care for Older People: Health Care of Older People Programme: Report of the National Audit of Continence Care for Older People (65 years and above) in England, Wales & Northern Ireland*, Royal College of Physicians, London, http://www.rcplondon.ac.uk/college/ceeu/coop/naccop_audit2005.pdf, accessed 13 January 2009.

Weisel, P., Norton, C., Roy, A.J. *et al.* (2000) Gut focused behavioural treatment (Biofeedback) for constipation and faecal incontinence in multiple sclerosis. *Journal of Neurology and Neuroscience Psychiatry* **69**, 240–243.

Wilson, J. (ed.) (1996) *Integrated Care Management: The Path to Success?*, Butterworth Heinemann, Edinburgh.

Index